AF372352

5livros.pt

RICARDO J. F. DIAS is a rehabilitation nurse, osteopath and trainer of health professionals and of alternative and complementary medicine therapists.

His passion is manual therapy, having developed, over the past 11 years, his own concept of therapy, working with body symbolism for physical, emotional, mental and spiritual treatment.

Among his training, the master's degree in sports sciences, coaching and the neurolinguistic programming master stand out.

In addition to his participation as a speaker in health and in alternative and complementary medicine congresses, his professional career includes 18 years of hospital experience and sports, as a nurse, 15 years as a vocational trainer, 11 years as an osteopath and as a life coach and 9 years as a manager of a health training company.

He is from Porto, Portugal, and it is through physical activity that he charges his energy. He is a fan of bicycle trips, with bags, and long walks, especially on the Santiago's Way or "The Way of Saint James".

You can find him at
www.touchingthehiddenyou.wordpress.com
or you can contact him directly using the email touchingthehiddenyou@gmail.com.
Facebook: touchingthehiddenyou
Instagram: touchingthehiddenyou
Amazon Author page: amazon.com/author/ricardodias
Goodreads: goodreads.com/ricardojfdias

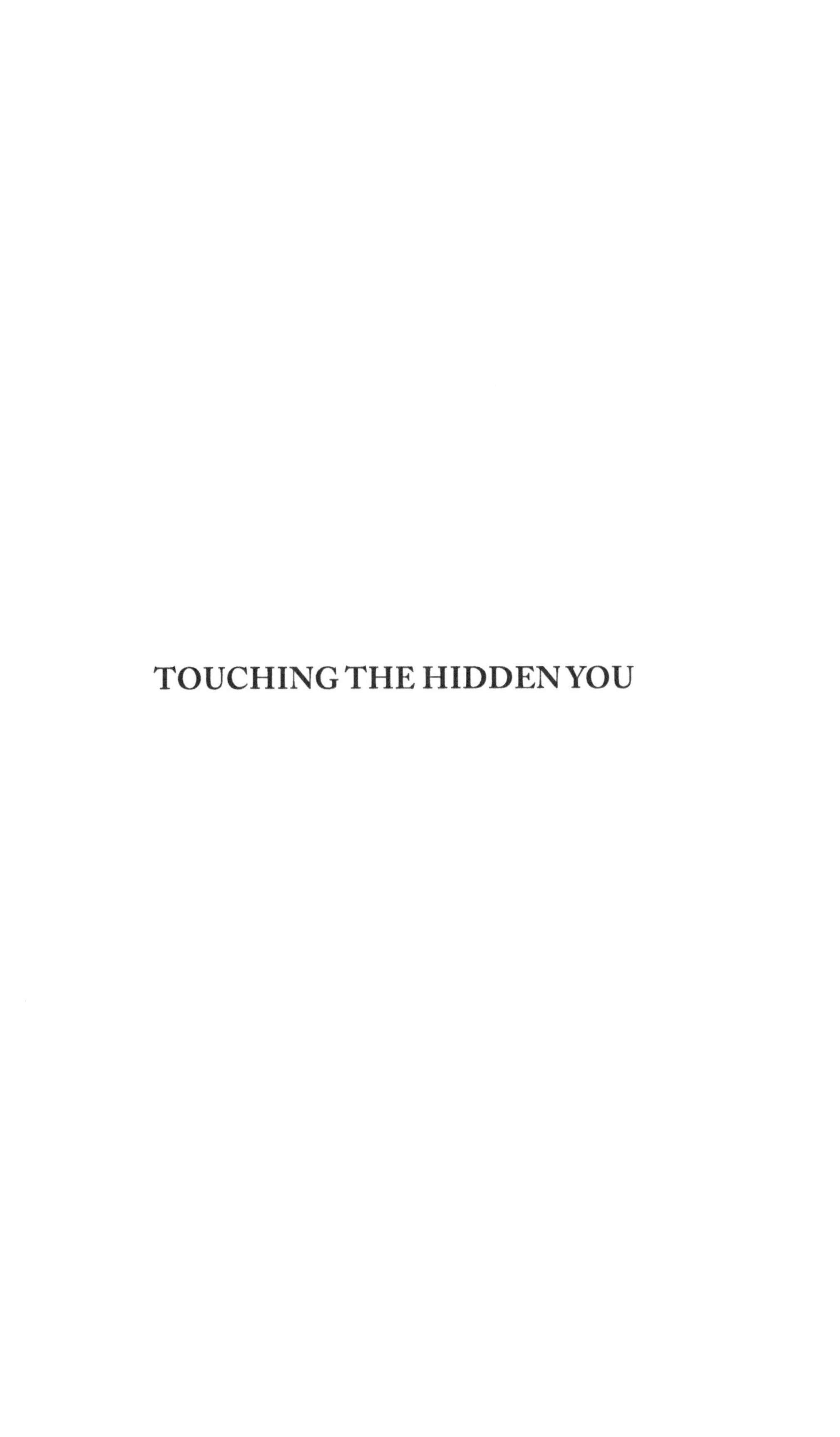

TOUCHING THE HIDDEN YOU

RICARDO DIAS

TOUCHING THE HIDDEN YOU

Therapeutic sessions that make us
question Life, Health and Disease

5livros.pt

Original title: Tocar no Eu Escondido: Sessões Terapêuticas que nos Fazem Questionar a Vida, a Saúde e a Doença
© Ricardo Dias, 2020
ISBN (Printed version): 978-989-782-018-2
ISBN (Digital version): 978-989-782-019-9
Originally published in Portugal, in 2020, by 5Livros.pt

1st Edition: March 2020
ISBN [Printed version]: 978-989-782-055-7
ISBN [Digital version]: 978-989-782-056-4

Categories in non-fiction:
1. Body, mind & spirit
2. Alternative & Complementary medicine

5livros.pt

Rua da Boavista, 719, 1.º T
4050-110 Porto
Telef.: 222 038 145
Tlm: 919 455 444
www.5livros.pt
info@5livros.pt

ÍNDICE

Dedicatory 9

Preface... 11

Acknowledgements 17

Chapter I 19
How things started and how health was so predictable 21
   Intuition 21
   INFJ personality 24
   Fate... 27
   Health. From the conventional.................................... 29
   ... To the "what the hell is going on here?" 43

Chapter II 53
And suddenly, everything I learned... faded away! 55
   The intention 59
   Case studies 64
      Susana, traumatic birth.. 66
      Susana's colleagues.. 70
      Sofia, my ex-libris... 77
      Pregnancy and childbirth 83
      Nuno, the rebirth and the "two faces"................. 95
      Cláudio and "messages from Beyond" 99
      The writing shoulder... 106

Health fair and the "restless hips" 110

Cristina and psychogenealogy 116

Headache and the right ovary 119

Ana, a right knee and a LED lamp 123

This is not the way you will communicate 127

Mental pop-ups 130

Pain in the legs and the burden legacy in childhood 132

Other cases 136

Chapter III **147**

From a free fall to a path of openness to understanding and acceptance   149

Learnings 149

Search for answers 150

The conventional approach 150

Osteopathy, sacro-cranial and fascial therapy 152

Coaching, neurolinguistic programming and hypnosis 158

Body language 163

Spiritism, psychogenealogy, exorcism and New Age 180

Ideomotor reflexes, applied kinesiology and radiesthesia ... 190

Others 196

Personal notes and guidelines 200

The infinitely big and the infinitely small 200

The mechanics of physical and emotional trauma 201

Ways of communication 203

Do not think. Wait! 205

Difficulties in communicating with the "non-conscious" or with the "parts" 206

Advice to health professionals 209

DEDICATORY

To my children

PREFACE

It took me three years to decide to write this book. It took me another four years to publish it. During this period, different feelings coexisted, in which the predominant one was frustration for not making my experiences public. Writing a book? Hmm! What an interesting idea! I never dreamed, nor did I think of writing a book. Why should I do it now? Do I have so much to share with someone? I feel average. From what I've learned throughout my life, the average person is not the one people talk about. Only the exceptional one. Those who stand out. Do I have that much to share that justifies writing a book? What do I want to show? Seeking recognition? Anything else?

My last seven years have been like this: an internal struggle that has completely changed my life. Maybe, I say, it was something "pre-written". Yes, destined to be that way. Walking along an almost certain path, passing through the tortuous path of constant doubts and suffering that is to become aware of my own ignorance and that everything I was taught could "not be quite like that".

This book will talk about my personal experiences (I can also say professionals) with people. Well, but this is common to all of us. We all relate to people! It is true. I will then talk about my personal experiences with people in the field of therapy. What therapy? For now, I will not go ahead with concepts of therapy or therapies. Just this idea: "therapy" as the answer we give to someone who seeks us to improve something in their health. I already know that, for the most critical, the concepts of "health" and "disease" are not clear. I leave it to your interpretation.

If you choose to read the book, if you are not bored with these first words, you will come across with concepts that can be controversial, subjective and misleading. Seven years ago, I wouldn't have thought to tell you this. These days, it makes perfect sense to me. This book results from a personal need to carry out a catharsis. So, believing (or not) in what I am going to tell you about my experiences, I will be at ease sharing what I found: a different world from the one I was told as a health professional. I will do a different analysis of the "human being", based on rich and complex areas such as medicine (as it could not be otherwise), psychology, psychogenealogy, neuroscience and (let's go to the prohibited concepts) alternative and complementary therapies (or unconventional therapies), religion, Spiritism, the occult, the phenomena of possession and exorcism and many other areas. Anyway, I believe that, in this line, many have already given up on reading and closed the book.

If you are one of those readers who keeps seeing what this gives, I present you a book that will talk about unconventional approaches to human health. I will not be concerned with clarifying or rambling on concepts. I will use mine, referring, as much as possible, to the sources from which I got some inspiration. There are many, now that I remember.

The book will talk about the way the "touch" led me to access information "secretly" hidden in each of us. That information you want to hide, but you can't. Or maybe you think you can do it. The "touch" that accesses the records of each one of us. Records that I am still not sure that belong only to our current earthly existence, or to past periods. Calm! I may be talking about "past lives", or "psychogenealogy", or just "mitochondrial memory", passed down from generation to generation. As I said earlier, the concepts are of little interest to me in this book. I am only interested in describing what I "saw", "heard" and "felt". It is a kind of "oral history", so used in gathering information, in qualitative research. Yes. I thought about writing this book only when I had done qualitative or quantitative studies on the topic. You know what? Probably, even when I was eighty years old, I would not be able to write a chapter, considering the vastness of the theories and concepts that I would have to analyse and the experiences that I would have to carry out. For now, the catharsis. To write the book. I will see what happens next. Although I already have an idea. I remember a professor's comment that I had during my specialization in Rehabilitation Nursing:

"Ricardo, I don't have a database that allows me to understand what you're saying.".

I am happy to have experienced "things" that I never thought existed. I am sceptical, very sceptical. Maybe that's why I question myself so much and question the world around me, sometimes becoming obsessed with subjects that interest me. I like to learn. I like to observe, test and create my own theories. Yes. We all have them. There's no need to get on the list of academic thesis creators and their hall of fame. Of course, it is in practice that we will analyse the impact of these same "theories", because in the dream plane nothing materializes. I am sceptical, as I was saying, but nothing prevents me from being fascinated by looking for what is "bizarre", "hidden", "esoteric" and "forbidden". In fact, the forbidden is very tempting. That forbidden, opened a horizon for which (I believe) I was destined. However, despite many positive points, it was a horizon that overwhelmed my life, to the point of no longer knowing "who I am", "what I do" and "where I am going to". I strongly believe that you have asked yourself several times with the same questions. Either you have questioned yourself, or you are questioning yourself, or, if not, it will be a matter of time before doubts begin to arise. For all those who have already overcome these existential dilemmas, my deep admiration and respect.

I consider myself an introspective and creative person who, above all, likes to create or transform. Let's say I have some difficulties in adapting to the institutionalized world, which preferentially values the "rational" and the "norm". Anyway, my "Shadow" tried to create or even transform what was within reach. Now that I know a little more about my numerology, many things make sense. No, I will not talk about numerology.

What did I have at my disposal before I came across with what led me to write a book? On the one hand, health training, as a nurse. On the other hand, the experience with people with disabilities or illness. Also, the experience of volunteering in various environments, in which I highlight the sports environment. Also, the experience as a trainer, which helped me to improve communication and study skills. The master's experience, in the systematization of thought and action. Most importantly: my training and experience in the field of manual therapy, with something as simple as... massage. Yes. As "simple" as "massage". A concept that, even today, I hear so vulgarly and that contains an indescribable potential. There it is... for those interested, right? I am interested. Perhaps therefore, with the natural evolution of my training in the field of manual therapy, I came across the "unspoken" of each one. What is this "unspoken"? For simplicity, in this book, I will use the concept of "non-conscious". Unlike "unconscious".

In short, the book talks about exactly this: the way I accessed the "non-conscious", with touch, having as somatic manifestations (visible, let's say) something that I had only seen in exorcism films. Yes. Yes. Yes. I could choose the words so as not to create "shock", or "indignation", or even "reluctance" to continue reading. No. The use of these words is fully conscious. The book talks about the path I took, from accessing other people's "non-conscious", just with my touch, to the emerging need to develop communicational skills, to use not only touch, but also the "word", to communicate. Communicate with what? With those "parts" of you, that you don't know they exist. Those "silent" and "hidden" parts that make life a hell. From simple manifestations such as pain, serious illnesses or repetitive life cycles. Repetitive cycles show us that there are life events that coincide with life events of our ancestors. They even coincide with age! It must be a coincidence, right? Wrong!

This is the field of study that I have been developing in recent years. Eight years ago, some of the therapeutic sessions were challenging for me to understand, which required some reflection and "return to earth". I needed to mature emotionally, and, in that sequence, I write this book, as a way of catharsis, to release my fears and face the fact that I still have much and much to explore.

There are several sources on which I rely for my actions and I know that it will be necessary to deepen each one of them. For now, I want to share my findings, realizing that, *per se*, the book will not have the impact of change that I would like it to have. It is the possible, now.

The book is structured in three chapters:

- Chapter I: How things started and how health was so predictable.
- Chapter II: And suddenly, everything I learned… faded away!

- Chapter III: From a free fall to a path of openness to understanding and acceptance.

Chapter I is a contextualization of my life until I was 28 years old. Despite being a chapter with a large autobiographical component, I consider it necessary to contextualize my view of health. You can skip ahead, but you will miss little details that can make a difference, for understanding Chapters II and III. In Chapter II, I describe the most remarkable experiences that made me question the concepts of "life", "health" and "disease". In Chapter III, I talk a little about each area of knowledge that was crucial to getting answers to my questions.

You will find many quotation marks. It is my style of writing, to draw attention to the concepts that I consider relevant. You will always find a word with quotation marks: "parts". This will happen because it is a concept that is quite comprehensive. Throughout the book, you will understand the scope of the term.

I wish you a good reading!

ACKNOWLEDGEMENTS

To those who created me difficulties, obstacles, doubts, suffering and despair. To those who kept me on earth and didn't let me fly.

To those who simply told me to go on.

CHAPTER I

HOW THINGS STARTED AND HOW HEALTH WAS SO PREDICTABLE

Year 2008. I was 28 years old and, just now, I understand that this date was a turning point in my life. It was not conscious. In fact, emotionally and even consciously, I can say that it was only in 2011 that I felt something different from what had happened to me until then: I felt that I "died" and that I "was reborn".

I will talk a little bit about my life until 2008. If you want, you can skip this autobiographical chapter. I understand it as necessary, to contextualize all the remaining chapters. In the sketch, the people closest to me, considered it expendable. After four years of reading this sketch, I continue to consider that this chapter is essential for the contextualization of the remaining chapters.

INTUITION

Until I was 28 years old, my life was like many others, but I highlight "that characteristic" that had been creating problems until I was 22: my "intuition". Talking about intuition is very interesting. At least two parts of me clash right away: the "angel" and the "little devil". The "angel" who tells me that intuition simply "IS" (and that of speaking only in "Being" and "Just Being" is a reason for discussions in various fields) and the "little devil" who says: "Hey! Ricardo. This is not scientific. Everyone knows that intuition only brings biased information.". Well, I confess that these disputes are still in my head today, but on a more peaceful level and in which both sides express themselves better and understand each other. In short, with less suffering for me.

Intuition. I don't know what you mean by intuition, but for me intuition is "to see beyond what is visible". It means having access to information that is not available in a "present" way. It is, in a way, foreseeing the future. In one way or another, intuition is present in each of us, but it was only at the beginning of my second decade of life that I realized that this intuition (which after all I was not even aware of it) was not developed in the same way in all people. Something that helped me remove some "weight", as I felt completely out of place in the face of "time" and "people". All excited and happy, I shared my "visions" with those around me: parents, friends, colleagues and other people. The result was similar: "What do you understand about this?", "You have no basis to support the statements!", "There you are making it up!", "That's what you say!". I heard other phrases, which I would prefer to omit. At this point, just an aside for a smile – ☺.

The truth is that I have always lived "out of place", feeling ridiculed and without being taken seriously. Even today, that happens. Probably the same will happen with what I write here so hard, thinking that I discovered gunpowder. I didn't discover it, but I may have found another way to light the fuse. What is certain is that, over the years, many of the "visions" that I had come true and several people came across me and recognized what I had transmitted to them. Interestingly, at that time, I was already talking again about my symbolic visions of the future and, once again, no one listened to me. Anyway! They say that "symbolism" is subjective and that everything we want fits there. I do not agree. The symbolism is quite accurate, especially when we talk about the symbolism of the body. Our body. But who am I to speak of symbolism? Other more accredited entities can help explain the "symbol" and its origins.

So, to put ourselves in context again, I was saying that my life was perfectly normal, apart from intuition, which, on the one hand, I discovered is a gift, but also the opposite: a headache! You are probably thinking about "curse". I prefer to call it "Shadow", according to an author I admire – Carl Gustav Jung.

I know now, since I mentioned Jung, that I have an INFJ personality. If you are a psychologist, I'm already waiting for you to put me on the Cross. Talking about Jung is like talking about "someone we should avoid". I believe this to be the case, as I continue to feel a lack of understanding of the scope of his work. Well then. Jung will have created a list of 16 personalities, in which, through various tests that I carried out, they all converge on one of these personalities. Not strangely, the rarest of all. Well, "Ricardo! Cool! You must be radiant! You are a rare person!". Apart from these comments that I know they exist, and that I even use them to play, the truth is that I learned a lot about myself from the analysis of this personality. Did I analyse myself only with the INFJ personality? Of course not. I used other means, other theories, and other approaches. But you know what? No matter how many laps it took, they all said similar things, whether through psychological tests, validated worldwide, or through numerology or even astrology. This is to emphasize that, for the essence of what I want to transmit, concepts are just concepts, so you are free to use them as you wish, provided that, in the end, you understand what I want to show and that you know how to get there on your own means. To introduce some of the most striking points of my life, I will start by explaining what the INFJ personality is, which I think I only discovered around my thirties. I will not go into more depth with Myers-Briggs personalities, based on Jung's study. Just talk a little about what INFJ is, to be able to frame my personal journey.

INFJ PERSONALITY

The INFJ personality is the rarest – some say two to three percent of the world population – of the sixteen personalities based on Jung. Of that three percent, probably only one percent will be male. INFJ combines characteristics that may conflict with each other but resulting in a person with exceptional qualities and equally exceptional weaknesses. Let's say INFJ will be the most like the "Superman" type, with "kryptonite" at his side, taking away his "powers".

In the "inner world", an INFJ person has two strong functions: introversion and intuition. In the "outside world", the person presents the functions feeling and judging. So, in general, we are dealing with a person who prefers to live in privacy, in solitude or in small groups of trust. The intuitive part makes the person more impulsive, acting according to "what I think is correct", based on "hunches". For people who need data to make decisions, intuitive people are considered impulsive and, to some extent, "crazy", for making decisions not based on facts, data or numbers. On the other hand, "intuitives" consider the "other side" as "down-to-earth", limited and not creative. The characteristic "feeling" is the weak point of the INFJ. It is true that they have an image of people who are cold, calculating, hard and unforgiving. The truth is different. Their reading of a person's "soul" allows them to obtain information that, many times, not even the person being analysed has any idea. They not only read the soul, but also the body. Very, very easily. The "feeling" is what allows to externalize the intuitive aspect: emotions, opinions, "visions" and the idea of the world. This is where things get complicated. In the world, INFJs are a minority. Most people use extroversion, analysis of hard data and thinking, as a way of establishing relationships. Most people will consider the INFJ person as soft, innocent, fragile, and easy to manipulate and change. They may even believe that they are achieving it. The "feeling" function will read all these intentions before they even become visible. In other words, even knowing that they are being deceived, the INFJ will (or will not) accept a certain submission, in order to remain part of a group. On the one hand, INFJs crave this belonging. On the other hand, they know that this is not what they want. The "vision" is often quite different from that which exists in the external world. As for the "judgment" function, it can be easily summarized in this way: if the INFJs have a keen intuition and an introspection that allows them to remain "in the rear", observing, analysing, taking notes and building theories, in addition to an exceptional ability to read a person's soul and body, then they will easily encounter communicational inconsistencies and act as a judge in a dry, hard and unforgiving way. They will do more if they realize that the inconsistency is conscious and used for evil purposes. They may also enter a spiral of suffering, if they realize that a person has high growth potential, but that they choose paths that will lead them in the opposite direction. It's devastating. It is also here that INFJs are easily deceived. When they trust someone's potential and they don't follow the path of spiritual growth. It is that the sense of personal integrity and value systems are untouchable. Combined with high perfectionism and a sense of "judgment", we have an uncompromising and hard person with himself and with others.

The INFJ personality is characterized by being idealistic and with a strong moral component. They are dreamers by nature and can realize their visions, with planned steps that cause great impact. If there are threats to this path of realization, or doubting their views, INFJ people will react impulsively and fight for the ideas they believe in. They are idealists, but they struggle to "prove their theory". They are charismatic, creative people, with strong communication skills, convincing and passionate, whose life mission is to help people and even take care of them. However, over the course of a lifetime, they alternate between opposites: from altruism (if a person is trustworthy), to more destructive selfishness (if the person has done something that has lost that same trust). They are tough critics (with themselves and others), but they tolerate criticism badly. They are very perfectionists. Criticism calls into question this same perfectionism. Something very common in INFJs is that they need to rest a lot and to have a private, silent and stimulus-free environment. Always in pursuit of the defence of a cause – idealism put into practice – they consume their energy very quickly, which often leads to depression.

At a professional level, they fall into professions that deviate from business standards, although they can also be very good in this area, especially as consultants, or "behind the scenes", or creative. They then fit into professions where there is some kind of "connection" with people, especially in their most holistic forms. It is common to find INFJs as consultants, psychologists, nurses, life coaches, "spirit guides", massage therapists or lawyers. All professions that allow the INFJ person to be in "control" of his life, will be fabulous. Although they do not like to "control" others, it is in leadership positions that they find their oasis, as it is the position that allows them to act following their heart, giving their "personal touch" and materializing their creativity and altruism. They are conflict managers by nature.

The INFJ personality is sensitive and mysterious, making it difficult to understand. Some well-known people, who are said to have an INFJ personality, are: Florence Nightingale, Carl Jung, Mahatma Gandhi, Fyodor Dostoiévski, Plato, Martin Luther King, Nélson Mandela, Al Pacino, Calista Flockart, Mel Gibson and Michelle Pfeiffer. If you must choose the Simpsons character, then that character will be the one represented by Lisa Simpson.

FATE

There are books that are marked in our lives. In saying this, I immediately must admit a major defect. I usually start reading a book and never finish it. In fact, I rarely finish it. It is as if a few pages were enough for me to understand the "global thing". When I reach the end of a book, it is a very good sign. It is a sign that I captured the information like a "sponge". One of those books is by John Parkin – Fuck It. Divine! Someone who captivates me to read from beginning to end, smiling from ear to ear, with a few laughs in between. An author who transmits knowledge in a way that only those with practical knowledge can transmit. With humour to the mix! At one point in the book, I read something that fascinated me and left me thinking. There is an analogy that the author makes with his childhood and with the carousels. The feeling of control in the carousels is fabulous. On their tracks, the carts turn to the left when we turn the steering wheel to the left. They turn to the right when we turn the wheel to the right. It is so fabulous to be in control! The author then proposes the possibility of doing something strange (perhaps unthinkable!): "What if the wheel is turn in the opposite direction to the curve of the carousel?". Well, here's the funny thing about the story: when you turn the steering wheel to the right side, the car continues to go to the left side and vice versa. So, what kind of control do we have?

If we think about this carousel analogy and carry it over to the whole analysis of our life, we will certainly notice that the supposed control we have over our life is illusory. It is true that we consciously make decisions and act according to our will, on the assumption of obtaining a certain result. But we all know that it is not so. We often hear: "You have to work, but you also have to be lucky!", Or "The less you want, the faster you will have!". So, what variable escapes us? Or the variables?

Fate. Someone calls it destiny. Just as the carousel has a line (trail) where little horses, boats and other entertainment so sought after by children (full of colour, sounds, movements and promises of a timed adventure), life also has this path already outlined for each of us. I know it is a controversial issue, questionable even to the marrow and everything. I'm not here to be part of a "Pro-Destination Party", but just to share that, recognizing a pattern in my life, I started looking for answers in books, in conversations, in films and in everything that "illuminated" me a little more. From the age of 22, my life seemed to be all stitched together, almost like editing a movie, with the sequences studied, the calculated dramas and the miraculous exits in a crisis. Very good! Of course, I also learned that life is made up of "ups and downs" and by living on a "high", for a decade, I also started a "depression" cycle, at the age of 31. I fully understand that in order to taste and value the sweet, it is necessary to try the bitter. Since the age of 31, I have been doing what I call "Valley of Shadows". More specifically, my "Shadow". Something that I hope is slowly disappearing and opening to a new cycle of growth.

Not before writing this book, as a catharsis.

HEALTH. FROM THE CONVENTIONAL…

I don't know if I'm more rational than emotional. I consider that I am both, without much distinction. On the one hand, intuitive and sensitive, on the other hand a "strategist", a "maker", capable of making the dream come true. The image that others have of me is probably more that of a rational person.

What led me to the health area was the fact that I had contact with health professionals in hospitals from an early age. My mother was a secretary in an Intensive Care service, and, for that reason, I learned about this environment from an early age. An environment that seduced me, it is true. Don't ask me why, although I remember that my childhood friend Filipe called me a hypochondriac. Whatever was a problem, there I went for my readings, in the health encyclopaedias, which my parents had on the shelves. There I tried to analyse the signs and symptoms and "fit them" in the most appropriate diagnosis. Many children would probably do so. But yes, I was obsessed with observing, theorizing, relating and solving. In this case, in the health area. Besides, and now that I remember some more things, it is true that observing, "dreaming" and "making" were common to many areas. In my backyard, I always turned to construction projects. Wood and earth were the elements that dominated my creations. Not forgetting the metal, present in the tools. Technology was also a "strong skill", with the first steps in broadcasting, with the creation of my "own radio" and a TV "channel". Too bad that few people had access to these childhood kidding.

I mentioned that what led me to the health area was my mother's influence, more "sensitive" than "objective". My father, on the other hand, a self-made man, was more objective. An avid reader, he worked in a Bank and always accompanied me (even if indirectly) in all my activities. I have always been encouraged to learn in several ways: learning languages, sports, technology and more. I was always busy and, despite that, encouraged. I was never the "excellence" student. "Medium" is the word that best suits. But now, aside, being average has been the subject of my analysis for many years. I conclude that it is good to be average. Even today, however, I keep a very vivid phrase in my head, from a professor I had during the curricular year of my master's degree in Sports Science, referring to the need to "specialize" in something, under the risk of not being good "at something":

"Duck. A duck knows how to swim. A duck knows how to walk. A duck knows how to fly. But it knows just a little of all of this. It doesn't compare to the dolphin's swimming. It doesn't compare to the horse's run. It doesn't compare to the eagle's flight. It is not a specialist in any of these activities.".

Well! Forgive me! Poor duck! As society is created, it is easy to criticize the "duck". On our planet, there are different species to live with. Choosing the "best" or "the worst" is, at the very least, anecdotal. They all have their role, even if it is not immediately visible. In the perspective of specializing in something, I agree with my teacher. But I also agree with the opposite. Having a comprehensive perspective of what is around us is important, at the risk of losing track of what we are doing. I also remember another statement that illustrates what I just said:

"The research is excellent to know a lot about the protein of the grasshopper's paw. But little of the grasshopper. ".

Of course, I'm not trying to convince – or irritate – anyone. Just to digress a little about the "extremism" that we like so much in our lives: "black-white" (forgetting the greys), "cold-hot" (forgetting the lukewarm), "good-bad", "science-religion". Basically, extremism only reflects the other side, in a kind of "Shadow Archetype" by Carl Jung. An extremism that makes us lose information and makes us more rigid and stuck to the matrix.

I felt that I lived between poles and learning to live among them. Trying to find a middle ground, with my own temperament, in the formation of character and a persona. My adolescence was a happy period. Very happy. Especially when I had the opportunity to live closely with sport, practiced by what we still call "people with disabilities". Aside from the linguistics we use, I lived closely with the personal dramas of these people and with the amazing way they saw, heard and felt the world. Deep down, what I found most was a deep feeling of "not feeling judgments" of any kind. There, as a practitioner, but also as a football and swimming monitor, I felt "Me". Far from the evaluation of the "excellent", "average", of having an X or Y brand car or wearing a Y or Z brand clothing. In fact, this was a personal development that brought me "value-added" for everything that would follow in my life – as a nurse, as a trainer, as a manager.

At the age of eighteen, I entered nursing, at a public school well known in the area: Escola Superior de Enfermagem de São João. On the one hand, a natural choice – the health area. On the other hand, a rational choice – I would have several professional opportunities. Yet another reason that it was to be a more practical than theoretical training, something that fits my way of being: "doing". I see now that nursing has allowed me to evolve in several fields because it has something that is unusual: it brings together several areas of knowledge and makes them practical. To a certain extent, it is the "duck" that I spoke about earlier. It encourages us to be versatile. To be creative. It also encourages us to maintain an "open view" about life. Over four years of training, at a time of great growth in class (nursing) recognition, I studied at a school that encouraged me to be objective, rational, but also human (what the hell is it to be "human"?), to question, to become more autonomous in my decisions and investigating as much as I could. To some extent, it is true, I started my profession by being more "technical". I believe that this happens in all professions, not just mine. Hence the famous book by Patricia Benner – "From Novice to Expert".

2001. End of the course. I started working at a General Hospital, the largest in the North of the country. At the same time, I continued my studies, to finish my graduation (at the time, I had a bachelor's degree and then one more year to finish my entire graduation), something that happened in 2002. I was lucky to work in an inpatient service that had children and adults, of both genders. It is not common! Nothing common. Children and adults, in the same service? Belonging to the same Unit, there was also an Intensive Care service.

This chapter is entitled: "How things started and how health was so predictable". It was something I felt until I was 28, during the first seven years of work: health was predictable. If someone likes numerology, then they can analyse the reason for the seven, in the context in which I move from "How things started and how health was so predictable" to "And suddenly, everything I learned... faded away!". In these seven years, I have invested a lot of time in work and training. As I write, I realize that the seven years were a short time, however highly productive. I learned a lot. "Health" is a very subjective concept, as are "human beings" and "life" itself. As health professionals, we are expected to know how to respond to requests for disease to treat or cure. That we also know how to prevent the appearance of diseases. Not only illnesses, but accidents – minor or serious. To some extent, all of us, as healthcare professionals, carry a responsibility to treat or heal people. Obviously, the term "carry" has not been used in vain and will probably make more sense at the end of this chapter and the next. Carrying the responsibility for healing someone... hmm... say... is asking too much. No? It is no coincidence that burnout exists in health professionals. Yes… yes… excessive hours of work also help. To be even more incisive, in the special case of nursing, there is still a low remuneration value, taking into account that we are given the responsibility to cure or treat sick people and those with very special needs (of total dependence on everything that is considered normal: eating, walking, going to the bathroom, reading a magazine, answering the phone, cooking, among others).

As a professional, directly or indirectly, an answer is expected from me. That I know how to act, through protocols and acts of evidence-based medicine. That I have "answers". Yes, until 2008, I believed that, good or bad, I had answers to give. Since then, a lot has changed.

Then returning to the seven years of "pure intensity", when health was so, but so predictable. Despite having started my profession to treat children and adults, something that enriched my global view of the "person", I recognize that it was the short time in Intensive Care that helped me to understand the body "mechanics". What a fabulous world, in which we have all the machines imaginable and unimaginable to support us to the "health" of the person. Ventilators for the person to ventilate (and breathe), perfusion machines to inject drugs of different "species and shapes" – to urinate more, to raise/lower blood pressure, to hydrate ourselves, to put us to sleep, to wake us up –, machines to "cleanse the blood" and replace the function of the kidneys, capsule cameras, to film the digestive tube, among many more. Ufff! Wonderful! What more could I want?

The little time I was in intensive care was well used. A lot of study, a lot of dedication and a new world to learn. I miss that time – just one year! My congratulations to those who have been working in Intensive Care for years. It was not because of my choice that I stayed only a year. At the time, circumstances beyond my control interfered with the path I was going to take: procedural errors in a public tender, judicial slowness and clientelism helped the process. The year I spent in Intensive Care was fabulous.

I was saying that it was a new world and that was the truth. With only one year of professional experience, as a nurse, I had never had contact with anything similar. Let's say that, at the time, I followed the more traditional paths in the stages of academic training: medical services, surgery, health centres and mental health units. I obviously must thank the team with whom I worked: they were demanding, good mentors and provided opportunities for growth. Being "below average" was very visible. I cannot say that there was the direct competition that you see in many workplaces. It was a happy competition, in which everyone wanted to apply what they knew best, in part to avoid "the jokes" of colleagues about something that went wrong (or less well).

Fortunately, I also had the opportunity to have training that was not accessible to most professionals (high costs) and to have met people with extensive experience in the area. I don't know what image you have of Intensive Care. The image I had was like "so much responsibility", "so much dependence", "so much work", "so much hardness", "so much machine", "so many details". Yes, I was right. In fact, it was necessary to work with systematization, concentration, efficiency and effectiveness (speed, no errors and obtaining results). What varies in relation to an inpatient service? Communication, no doubt. Most of the time – I dare say in ninety percent of cases – people are in what is called "induced coma".

Or they are really in a coma. So, if you think that communication is just talking, this would not be a service where you would like to work. Obviously, we did, but mainly with families, which was not easy either. In Intensive Care, I learned to work fast, to save lives. It would have been useful if I had also worked in Emergency services, but I confess that it was never an area that seduced me. I learned many technical procedures, I attended many types of exams and, with these, I learned to know the human body, in a very physical way. When I talk about "physics", I mean understanding the mechanisms that make us ventilate, making exchanges between oxygen and carbon dioxide, managing those same changes with those that occur at the renal, hepatic level, and so on. To some extent, as professionals, we take care of the functioning of a person's body. Believe me. There is a lot to do. I confess that what gave me the most pleasure was to analyse the ventilatory and renal function parameters and to anticipate the outcome. Working with ventilators and hemodiafiltration machines was what I loved to do. I took advantage of my night shifts to study, while analysing the monitors of each of the six people hospitalized in the service. It was not very large, compared to other Intensive units. Colours and sounds. Typical of a Unit of this kind. Colours of all kinds, for all types of vital parameters. Sounds from ventilators "blowing" air into the lungs, sounds of alarms, sounds that were indicating normalcy and a unique feeling of being in a quiet environment (at night and when everything was going well).

When I finished the nursing course, I started the interesting journey in the world of "touch". My father recognized in me the need for manual work – "doing with my hands" – and enrolled me in a massage course. I still think about how a "simple" massage course brought me here. Over the past few years, I realized that, in fact, massage therapy is a profession of choice for me: contact with people, close contact with emotions and with their most intimate and protected side. It was a short course, but it allowed me to absorb the information like a "sponge". In addition to my existing knowledge, acquired in the nursing course, it was easy to follow the theoretical approach. Still, I was fascinated to study the history of massage, its components, the different techniques and temporal and cultural contexts. What fascinated me most was the practice and, naturally, motivated, I committed myself to learn the most and to do perfectly what they taught me.

I finished the course in December 2001, as I recall, although I only received my certificate in March 2002. During this period, between December and March, I took the opportunity to take the "Trainer's Certificate" course, which would also be fundamental in my professional career (to teach in Vocational Training). Later on, I will talk about the importance of this training, to justify that much of the knowledge that makes me write this book was only possible because I had at my disposal a formidable group of people – especially trainees – who agreed to help me in many of my "experiences". Most of them with reach above my expectations. But let there be no mistakes! For fifty percent success, we have just as many failures. In April 2002, the school I graduated from contacted me. As I was the best in the class, they were contacting me because an Ayurvedic therapy centre needed a therapist and was willing to train him to work in the field. I accepted the challenge that was opening and went to an interview at that centre. I got scared when I entered. I don't know if "scared" was the real reaction I had. Fright, fear, amazement, I'm not sure. The centre was just fabulous. If you ask me to describe it, I am afraid of falling short of expectations. In fact, something I haven't mentioned yet: I tend to be very succinct and direct. I like to "digress", "theorize", "philosophize", but I am very synthetic, and I have difficulties in translating into words everything that goes through my head. My mind is a whirlwind of ideas and relationships between them, which become more visible when I do something. I say execute, perform and not "speak". Therefore, writing this book is also a catharsis in that respect. **Speak!** (or write).

To speak of this centre, even today, after seventeen years, is indescribable. A centre that we cannot say was "big", but it was also not "small". We are talking about a space of about 7535 ft², divided into three floors, decorated essentially with Palo-Santo and marble. Quiet, with soft music – which reminded me a little of Tibetan music – and an odour that I could not attribute to anything I had already smelled, certainly coming from the different Indian oils and teas that existed in the place. The hall was spacious, with a reception area that, right behind, had a staircase that led up to a floor where most therapies were performed. Common spa, where no client crossed, because all the therapists were articulated so that it didn't happen, just to allow more privacy and silence on the premises. With that, yes, many of the treatments lasted longer than expected, which made the place itself more intimate to obtain the relaxation that was so desired. The treatment offices were fabulous and perfect, considering everything I had studied in the massage course. Quiet, welcoming, indirect lights, Palo-Santo tones, with the orange light of lit candles, reddish marbles, wooden tables, towels, oils, *pinda sweda* and *shirodhara* equipment. I entered a new world. I trained with an Indian therapist, from whom I learned little, partly because of the language barrier and the complexity of Ayurveda. Still, with a lot of study, I learned a few things about Ayurveda, namely some of the most common therapies, equipment and consumables used and the concepts of *doshas* – *Vatta, Kapha, Pitta*. I never learned Indian pulse diagnosis. Unfortunately. The centre also had a lower floor, with more changing rooms and offices.

It also had Turkish bath cabinets, which we could use at the end of a working day. In general, I can say that I lived in paradise: SPA in all its splendour. It is true that there was no water treatment with swimming pools, waterfalls, water jets and thermal waters. I couldn't be too demanding. The existing conditions were fabulous. They transported us out of Porto (the city where I live and where the therapy centre was located), in Portugal, in the blink of an eye.

Working at this centre marked me by the visible cultural differences. Our target audience was the middle-upper and upper classes. We served Portuguese, but also many foreigners. Here, cultural differences began, to which I was not yet accustomed, especially related to nudity. For most foreigners, massage treatment was something normal and routine in their lives, with common spas (without gender division) and complete nudity. I confess that, at 22, it was not nudity that worried me. It was what was inherent in it and which I intuitively perceived easily: the absence of touch in people's daily lives. The absence of affection, caresses and a sense of belonging. There, in that space, frequented by both men and women, what was most sought after was a space where touch was possible, without judgment, without great conversation. Just feel the naked body, to be touched. Many of the people who frequented the space came from the corporate and political areas. Wives of influential people in society – often absent from home – were enough. Lonely travellers, ditto. Looking more clearly, after these seventeen years, I would say that nudity was not as natural as many people believed. I would almost say it would be a paradoxical reaction. On the one hand, the conscious choice of the integral nude, giving the image of: "Yes. It's my option. I am a safe person.". On the other hand, shyness towards the therapist and the inability to fully relax. I wish I knew what I know today. It would be a fertile field to explore the bodily symbolism that I will talk about in Chapter III. I would summarize nudity to something like this: "Here is my body. I show it to you. I let you touch it, but please understand it.". I speak of nudity, from a personal and professional perspective, which has its typical "filters". Naturally, it was important to analyse other concepts of nudity, from an artistic perspective – drawings, nude photography, sculptures – but also anthropological. Through his training in zoology, Desmond Morris was an author who brought important knowledge to the analysis of human beings. In a humorous way, I would say.

Nudity. How can you perceive so much of a person. How so cunningly we hide behind clothes, accessories and modify all the perception that others have of our real "me". The truth is that this "real me" is purely conceptual. There will be no "me" or "real". There may be several "selves" and reality is built through interpretations that we make. I will not go much further in this field. Many "weighted" authors talk about this topic. Let me just speak freely of the interpretation that "I" give to "things" and the result that I obtain in practice. Nudity. The body transmits to us everything we want to hide. Tell us what we don't want to say. Tell us who we are, even if that is not at all what we think we are. Of course, we need to have new "glasses" to see, hear and feel what's in front of us. I remember a funny moment that happened with a colleague of osteopathy. Brazilian, a "flirt guy", sadly confesses to me:

"I don't know if I did well to take the osteopathy course. Before, I looked at women's butts and seduced me. Now, I look and see only misalignments and say to myself: 'Hey boy! That iliac is misaligned! You have to align!'.

I was saying that if it was today, I would have a fertile field to analyse the symbology of the human body in its best form of evaluation: naked. The truth is that the short time I was in this therapeutic centre – due to poor management of the place, I chose to leave – helped me to know a part of society that I did not know.

Typically, people often say that I can't stand still and that's for some reason. In mid-2003, I left the centre of Ayurveda and set out to create a massage service for athletics events in my city. For that, I contacted the organization that organized this type of events, here in Porto. Today, it is the largest organizer of athletics events in this city. At the time, it would already be, but never with the scale it has today. Let's say it was a symbiosis. I was interested in continuing to learn manual therapy and gaining experience and contacts. The organization was interested in creating a service that, until then, was practically non-existent in sports events: sports massage. New challenge. Working with organizations related to sport was something that motivated me. Since childhood, the taste for sport had always existed, having been a swimming and martial arts athlete and, in a playful way, I dedicated myself to athletics. As a teenager, I was also a soccer and swimming monitor for athletes with mental disabilities and cerebral palsy, at Futebol Clube do Porto. I remember those times with nostalgia.

It would then be necessary to combine the professional aspect and the passion that was beginning to grow for manual therapy, with the support of health to sportsmen. The beginning was interesting. The first athletics event that I supported would have around 2000 participants and, with the help of a colleague of mine, from the massage course, in a 3x3m tent, with two massage tables, there we were assisting the people who were in line. Obviously, the goal would be just to help the recovery, to give some sense of "we are here", to diminish any pain that existed and to increase the general well-being of people. Being around ten minutes with each one, there is no time for more. From then on, the challenge was greater:

how could I maintain support for sporting events, with only two people, since it was on a voluntary basis and that few would accept those conditions? Mainly, I was moved by the passion for learning and the desire to contact people, obtaining instant feedback on my work – "did it work?", "did it improve?", "did it get worse?". At the same time, other questions arose: "how can I treat that?", "how?", "what do I need to learn more?". I couldn't demand that others join me for the same ideals.

Fate or destiny. I already talked a little about the concept of fate. A kind of carousel trail that, regardless of all the efforts we make to turn to the "right", will have reserved other types of paths, such as the "left". Carl Jung has an interesting (and different) destination concept:

"Until you make the unconscious conscious, it will direct your life and you will call it fate.".

I was then in a phase of life when I wanted to continue supporting sporting events, but I knew that I would need a bigger infrastructure and more people. Well, for a few years now, there's been a lot of talk about the "power of attraction." In this case, it might as well apply. What I needed... I had. Was it my thought? The fate or destiny? The trail that was (is) already created for me to go? One thing was certain. In my life, it seemed that everything happened in a synchronized way (synchronicity). In 2002, along with hospital work, I invested time and money in knowledge – courses, congresses, workshops and others. I was motivated and everything was new. I absorbed knowledge at great speed. I continued my training in electrotherapy, in joint mobilizations and similar subjects, to be able to work as a physiotherapy assistant. Naturally, I was not interested in going to work for a physiotherapy clinic, but rather to complement my nursing training with knowledge that did not exist in the training plan. That motivated me, of course! In this training, I was very disappointed with the "system", due to a poorly prepared trainer, who did not encourage the search for knowledge. In fact, I may even say that she destroyed it. Even with evidence, from different sources, she refused to accept the "evidence".

Apart from the case with the trainer, I learned interesting things that piqued my curiosity even more. I also had the opportunity to meet interesting people, one of whom showed interest in accompanying me to the second athletics event that I was going to support, in December 2003. At this time, I got the sponsorship of two massage tables, which I needed for supporting the athletes. Still, there were some problems: growing interest in sports massage by the athletes; need to improve logistics; need to have more professionals to accompany me. Well, it came on purpose! I was receiving my Trainer's Certificate (maybe in October 2003) and receiving an invitation to teach at the institution where I had taken the massage course and the physiotherapy assistant course. They were looking for a nurse, for teaching healthcare in sporting! Perfect! From this moment on, with all my investments going perfectly (okay… I am envious of those young people who create an *app* and earn millions in a matter of minutes) and three months later, another invitation arrives to be a teacher of massage therapy. Interestingly, there were not so many people with that certificate (mandatory for professional/ vocational training) and with training in massage. Even if there was, they apparently had no interest in accepting it. For me, it was an opportunity, to be able to combine areas I love: health, vocational training and sport.

It was in this context that, for three years, I grew up at various levels. Doing things I liked and gaining skills, especially in terms of interpersonal communication, conflict management, socialization, and much more. Without thinking too much, I got what I needed. I continued to support sporting events – more and more and bigger – having fifty massage therapists available for the first time in an event that was "only" the first marathon in the city of Porto. Trainees, former trainees and an energy and passion in their massage training, at the same time that I started to create my path in team management, organization of health support for athletes and everything that is inherent to it: sponsorship, contact with organizations, specific training for the sports, with massage and first aid (essential for my goal). Tired, but motivated, as always!

From 2001 to 2006, I summarize my life in just one paragraph: hospital work, work as a healthcare trainer and continuous personal studying. "Health" was an objective, somewhat predictable concept. My personal path was predictable. Anyway, everything seemed predictable. In that predictability, I entered the osteopathy course. In all the sense it made. Until I found unpredictability.

... TO THE "WHAT THE HELL IS GOING ON HERE?"

July 2008. With my touch, the girl lying on the massage table loses voluntary control of the body. The body enters a typical tetanic position. The neck looks like it's going to break. It's bright red, the veins look like they're going to burst. The clenched teeth, the red face, the contracted body, practically with few body areas resting on the massage table (how is that possible?). Groans that look like anger. Anger or aggression? I don't even know. What the "hell" is happening? More important than that! How do I stop what I triggered?

Before I continue to explain this situation, I need to explain that, with the natural "flow" of my training and the interest for manual therapy – massage – it made perfect sense to continue my studies with osteopathy. This interest had been going on for some years, but the truth is that the lack of standardization of the contents taught by the schools of that time and the doubt that it cast on the quality of these same programs meant that I only started the respective course in December 2007. At that time, osteopathy was not the most popular course of non-conventional therapies, compared to acupuncture and homeopathy. Many lobbies in the middle influenced the credibility of existing courses, channelling training to only a couple of institutions. Something that fortunately came to change, with the recent alteration of the law on non-conventional therapies, which now have uniform training and conditions for the practice of the profession.

I remember being at work and receiving a call to inform me that there would be a course to start soon – the first edition – and to probe my interest in attending it. My first question was not as obvious as you might think. "Who gave you my number?", I asked, already suspicious. Well, after all, everything was apparently fine. It had been a massage therapist with whom I had worked at the Ayurveda centre. "Explain to me how the course is going to unfold and what areas it will address.", I continued. The conditions were explained to me and I was pondering the matter. There would be a face-to-face session to present the course, to which I went, in order to "feel" the environment. It is true that, in general, I was interested in the course, although I recognized some (serious) flaws in advance, which I would easily overcome with my academic training and professional experience. Price? Expensive! But willing to make the investment. Despite being young – 27 years old – and working only six years ago, I could feel satisfied with the life I was leading, although it was a critical time in my life (yes, I know... so young and with so many existential dilemmas), with cleavages at the professional level.

I was pleased to be working in a public hospital and the job security it could bring. On the other hand, as a vocational trainer, I was going through a time when I had a lot of training in massage therapy and training in sports. Everything I loved. I was in contact with several people, outside the scope of health, I had finished my master's degree in Sports Sciences and had "disconnected" from the athletics events organizing company, due to lack of recognition and personal saturation (I was tired of doing the same thing). I started to collaborate with other sports organizations, who expressed their interest in having me as a collaborator. I continued to do something I liked, but with organizations that gave me more recognition and appreciation for the sports massage work I was doing. Between 2006 and 2007, it was a time of tension at the personal and professional levels. The "mirror" has these things, because the "Shadow" accompanies the growth of the "Light" (knowledge). These moments of tension boil down to bullying and professional instability. All the changes that were happening were making me feel "stuck between the cross and the sword", so I decided to come up with an "idea" that I already had: create my vocational training company. It would be a challenge. I had no training in management. I had no family members with experience in creating and managing companies, but I felt I could do it. After several months of walking back and forth, studying business plans and other bureaucratic matters, I decided to move on to the creation of my own company. Something I gave up in November 2007. Because of the fear of failure. When I say I gave up, I really did it. I accepted that I would never be able to do it. Until the beginning of January 2008, after a month without thinking about anything. With an unusual energy, I was thinking that I was going to accomplish it, breaking all family cycles and risking. Everything could go wrong, putting my savings at risk. But I had unusual energy and intuition. It was to be done. And so, it was. I created the company on February 22, 2008.

So, the osteopathy course came at this time. Hospital work, training, company, course and finances tight. My mind was flowing like never. Intuition likewise. Motivation also. I was unaware that after three years I would enter a "descending" cycle, unprecedented. Almost as if it were the compensation/ balance, of these wonderful times that I was living. The osteopathy course opened practical horizons for me! Having osteopathic knowledge helped me in the therapeutic evolution, namely in sporting. Fabulous, no doubt. If you know little about osteopathy, let me clarify the concept. Osteopathy is a therapy that uses bone manipulation as the foundation. In general, the alignment of certain bone structures will contribute to the overall alignment of the body. It will tend to the so-called homeostasis and balance. Of course, these are general concepts and it is not my intention to make a compendium or treatise on osteopathy. Osteopathy uses massage a lot (something I love) and more incisive techniques, called *thrust*. So far, nothing new.

Health remained predictable! "I handle this bone here and it will have results there.".

In the field of osteopathy, there are three views: structural osteopathy (more physical, more contact with the skeleton); visceral osteopathy (organ manipulation, via physical or "energetic" interventions) and energetic osteopathy. Let's be frank. How many energy books are there in bookstores? Many! How many try to explain the energy? Many! How many try to prove that it exists or that it does not exist? Many! So, what the "hell" is energy? Everything sparked a lot of interest in osteopathy, but nothing as much as the concept of "energy". It was here that the turning point in my life began. Without me realising it.

Sacro-cranial therapy. A concept created by Upledger. Basically, sacro-cranial therapy assumes that we all have a "subtle" rhythm in the body, unlike any other that we know, such as heart or lymphatic rhythm. Sacro-cranial presupposes a CSF rhythm (cerebrospinal fluid), a fluid that protects our central nervous system. Any disturbance at this rate will lead to physical and emotional problems. What problems? The literature will spell out several problems, from a headache to depression. Nothing objective, for the most sceptical and rational. Therapy assumes that this cycle has "flexion" (opening) and "extension" (closing) movements. Someone with a cycle that is too "flexed" may be overconfident, perhaps arrogant, overbearing and possessive. On the contrary, a person in extreme "extension" may be a depressed and melancholy person. It is not for me to dwell on the sacro-cranial theory, but to take the concepts that raised questions and that led me to incredible experiences. One of the interesting moments of sacro-cranial learning was the fact that we had to stand still. Standing still? Yes. Stopped. The more still we were, the better. The less pressure we put on the person, the better. The reference was simple: "Your hands cannot weigh more than a €1 coin!". Or would it be 50 cents? I don't remember exactly. But as I didn't have a device at my disposal to accurately assess the pressure I was exerting, the concept was simple: "Ricardo, do little or no pressure.". Good. Here, in fact, the concept was interesting. Applying little pressure just to "feel" what we were not used to "feel", daily and even as therapists – even coming from the field of manual therapy. "Feel what?". This question has been on my mind for several days. "What do I have to feel?". The truth is that I was looking for "nothing". I had to feel something, but I didn't know what. To help, my teacher was a motivator: "It may take two years to start feeling.". Fabulous. It can take up to two years before I start to feel anything, but without really knowing what. For our exercises, the scheme was simple and even used a lot in different contexts: we experienced the "subtle touch" in all our colleagues. A "round" for some. A round for others. The initial exercise was simple. It was to train the so-called "expansion O". What is "expansion O"? The "expansion O" is very similar to what the Japanese comic book hero Son Goku was adept at doing: *Kame Hame Ha* (balls of fire and energy). The concept was very simple: I had to put my hands on certain places of the person's body, I had to imagine a "ball of energy" between my two hands and then I would have to wait for something to happen. "Here we go again.", I thought. I had already felt "magnetism" in certain training exercises for massage therapists. I had already felt my hands as if they were connected by magnets – not very strong, but perceptible. But it had been a long time since I had felt something similar. There were certain areas where we put our hands that, interestingly, were like the areas where we put our hands in reiki. Hence many people ask me: "Are you doing reiki?". "No, I'm not doing reiki.". I will talk about reiki, but only in Chapter III. The truth is that I was responding that way out of anger. Anger at not knowing what I was doing, or what to call it. If reiki was what people understood, then that's fine... I was doing reiki. Concepts, nothing more than concepts and drawers. It is part of human nature that we want to shelve everything, label everything, name everything, order everything.

Now, the "expansion O" was carried out in several areas of the body: head, shoulder girdle, solar plexus, navel, thighs, knees, legs and feet. The hands were placed so that we could imagine a "ball" between the hands. There we went from colleague to colleague, experiencing the subtle touch. No results. Nothing at all. I just felt "nothing". The "nothing" is in itself an "existence". The brain needs to create an image, a feeling, a sound, anything that represents "nothing". For some, it is a white space, for others, a black space, for others it is silence. The "nothing" differs between all of us. The "nothing" for me was the frustration of not feeling the energy ball appearing in front of my eyes and being able to make a *Kame Hame Ha*. There I was changing partners again and… behold… nothing again. Only after some time, after having gone through half a dozen colleagues, did something different arise. The colleague to whom I was doing the "expansion O" got up from the massage table, looked at me seriously, and whispered to me: "You, of all those here, will be going far. You don't have an idea of your potential!". Well… joy…! Finally I had my ego (and when I speak of ego, I speak of that conscious, rational, earthly part, which is afraid of everything, which puts obstacles in everything and anything else, that part that makes you retreat when you feel you must move forward) petted. How good it feels to be "Special". My question is: "Special" in what? I would rather not have heard anything than to have a supposed compliment or statement that made me "vain", but that only brought more obstacles than answers.

A month later, I started to realize what he had said to me. At that moment, I just kept that idea in my head. It was time to switch roles and I was going to receive "expansion O". Emotion! What would I feel? Was I going to be "Enlightened" in any way? Well… no. I felt practically nothing, with anyone. Except for that colleague of mine, who barely put both hands on my chest, the words could not describe the feeling: I was losing control over my body and emotions were trying to spring up. With strength. No, I didn't cry. I didn't even feel like crying. Just laugh. Laughing out loud. I was trying to control myself, but I just wanted to laugh. Laughing madly, as I haven't done in years. Genuine laughter, coming from I don't know where. From my current experience, I know that behind the laughter, like onion skin, come other "skins", with different emotional charges and with different physical manifestations. Some, worse than exorcism sessions. In my case, no. Just laugh and laugh. It was a feeling like what had happened a few months before, when, for the first time, my teacher manipulated my cervical vertebrae. Especially C1. I still remember it well. A Saturday afternoon, around 5pm. A strong "crack", a burning sensation throughout the body. Intense heat. I went home, had dinner and went to sleep. But I spent the night laughing compulsively. Fantastic. An emotional release caused by cervical manipulation! I went to the course the next day. Still laughing.

I remember that this "expansion O" session took place before we went on vacation. So, we would be at the end of June or July 2008. In the meantime, I was still interested in learning more and experimenting with someone. To put it in context, at this time, I already had my vocational training company, in which the bet was placed on training health assistants, but also with a bet on massage therapy courses, postural re-education and similar courses. At the same time, I was also a trainer at another training centre, teaching massage therapy. So, to some extent, I had the ideal conditions to practice and test my knowledge. I had trainees willing to serve as "guinea pigs" and to accompany me in the new "theories" that I had brought. I don't remember the day, unless it was late July 2008. I only remember the hour: 12:50. I had finished a massage class and was explaining the new concepts I was learning, namely "expansion O". A woman expressed an interest in experimenting, and I volunteered to do a demonstration. She lay down on the massage table, while the rest of the trainees packed up their things to leave. I was still talking to them, smiling, when I put my hands on the chest area, as I had learned. "I'm going to imagine the energy ball in my hands.", I thought. I didn't even have time for that. I was still talking to some trainees, when I started to feel my hands shaking. It was not me. It was her body that was moving. But it was strange. Everything was strange. It was not something I had ever seen. Even now, it will be difficult for me to explain in words what I felt at that moment. The woman – I'm going to call her Susana – was still talking to me, but her body seemed to be reacting independently to her will. This was quite noticeable in her face. Some fear, I believe. It wasn't just hers. It was also mine. I was focused on everything that was happening in front of me. What I was seeing, what I was feeling and what I was hearing. There is no doubt of what I will say: I had only seen similar things in exorcism films. The body started to become tense, to adopt typical tetanic postures (in which the contraction is so violent and involuntary that only the heels and the head are supported on the ground), the upper limbs to rotate externally, the hands to accompany the movement and to do a forced extension. If this was already frightening, it scared me more to feel the chest moving in the opposite direction to the abdomen. It was as if something was moving inside Susana. In fact, everything seemed to move in a chaotic way. If we are made of "pieces", well… this was a moment to see each one moving independently. What scared me the most was what happened next: the extreme extension of the head, the thyroid cartilage wanting to "go up" (Susana was lying down and, seen from the side, was the perspective I had at the moment), the veins becoming protruding, skin turning red, muscle contractions increasing. Teeth clenched and groans of anger or aggression. I don't even know yet what that would be.

First reaction: fear. Fear of not understanding what was going on. Fear of not knowing how to stop those reactions. "What the hell is going on?". In fact, more important than that: "How do I stop this?". Not knowing how, I intuitively just thought, "Stop". I didn't verbalize. I just thought. What is certain is that it stopped. Some trainees looking at me. I was looking at them. Silence. Until then, everything seemed predictable and logical. Until that moment. From there, I had to admit the hypothesis that everything I had learned, until then, could be (euphemistically) out of date.

CHAPTER II

AND SUDDENLY, EVERYTHING I LEARNED…
FADED AWAY!

The title of this section reveals my deepest feeling: from that session with Susana, everything I had learned, until then, was seriously questioned. I had heard of many therapies related to energy and its effect on people. I had never heard of anyone having similar reactions to this. Yes, there is a book that talks about something similar, which is the book "Reconnection", by Eric Pearl. I find common points in the "findings", but from the little I read – I admit that I didn't read the whole book – I find differences in the theories behind the practice. My father says to me:

"There are as many therapies as there are therapists.".

It is true. Each of us, with our filters, apprehends the world in our own way and, obviously, also we act on our own way. It is an identity that sets us apart from the rest. One of my characteristics is to love the "hidden" and to love challenges and new things. I love being able to explore the "hidden", which is "beyond" what is taught to us in conventional ways. What that moment with Susana provided me with was one of those opportunities: studying what I call "I don't know what". The expression may generate indignation in the most "learned", but certainly, in the context of this book, they have already given up on reading it and have already classified it as a tremendous "****".

Undoubtedly, that moment marked a separation from my linear idea of health, from my current (much wider) idea of what health and disease is. The experiences that resulted from it: accessing non-conscious "records" through touch; visualizing somatic manifestations worse than scenes from exorcism films (I admit that I didn't see anyone walking around the ceiling, as if they were a spider, or turning their heads 360º); feeling "parts" of the body moving according to my "intention"; talk (yes, literally) with illness; negotiate the "cure" and much more. All formidable experiences. No doubt. Above all the show-off experienced, there is a lesson that remains and that I have shared since then with all my graduates and people with whom I have the opportunity to talk about topics such as soul, spirit, emotion, body, health and disease:

As health professionals, we are trained to respond to people's illnesses. In a way, we are the healers. With what I experienced, I realized that my role was more of a mediator, than a healer. There is an "inner wise man" in each of us, who will know what we need. If there is a "cure", it is because there is permission from this "wise man" for me to intervene. Not because I want to, but because I am authorized to do so.

The role of the health professional is the topic that still causes me the most difficulties. What is expected of the health professional? Do you know? I don't know it anymore. Are we expected to have answers for the cure? Healing of what? Physical? Emotional? Mental? Spiritual? Energetic? Right now, not being able to interact with you, I just ask you to ask the following question: "What do I expect from a health professional?". More specifically, what do you expect from a nurse (as in my case?). The typical answers? Active listening? Understanding? To be "sweet"? Anyone who has technical skills? Someone that is "scientific"? What is "health" for you? What is "disease" for you? Let us return to the classic philosophical questions: "Who are we, where did we come from and where are we going?". These are questions that I ask, but for which I do not have the miraculous answer to give you. The most I can do is to put you questions and explain how I solved some of the doubts that I found.

Imagine this scenario. You can touch a person. In just a few seconds (or a few minutes) that person loses voluntary control of the body. The body starts to react only to what you ask, such as: "raise your arm", "lower your arm", "self-correct the injury", "write me what you need". How does it feel? I will repeat it again, in case it went unnoticed. I am proposing a scenario in which you have Mrs. Y in front of you. Let's say she has a shoulder pain. Without speaking, I repeat, without speaking and just touching that person, you can communicate with her body, making it move according to your thoughts – a movement that is independent of the will of Mrs. Y. In fact, she doesn't even hear you! How can she even imagine what's on your mind? How do you feel to see the body reacting according to your thinking? I do not imagine your answer, nor will I'll try to guess it. I do share what I felt, over the course of several sessions like this case: amazement! I still feel it in every session. Stupefaction. It is obvious to me that I am in one of those phases of learning which is "I don't know that I know.". As much as things come to me intuitively, the truth is that, since 2008, the struggle has been to understand what I do, in order to be able to replicate or teach others. One thing is certain! It is teachable, as I have had several cases in which I managed to get others to have similar results. It is also true that the more resources we have at our disposal the better. Learning is continuous and, over the past few years, I have felt the need to answer many of my questions. I immediately recognize the biggest problem of all: how to deal with somatization and what does it mean? I will clarify these concepts. "Somatic" is the "visible" form, quickly identifiable by several people. "Somatic" is how "something" is "manifested". In this sense, we have many forms of manifestation. Everything about us is somatic! The way we speak, how we walk, how we write, how we interact with others. In health, we use the terms "psychosomatic" to refer to problems of a "psychological" source in "physical" and "somatopsychic" to the way physical problems affect the psyche. In just one sentence, I referred to terms that can *per se* give rise to several term clarification articles. As I said earlier, it is not my intention to dwell on concepts.

Initially, my problem was dealing with the somatic reactions that were triggered by my touch. Imagine that you have a "healthy" person in front of you, lying on the couch and that, when you touch him/her lightly on the head, for ten minutes, he/she starts to stop breathing and become white (or purple). Interesting? Spooky? For me, both. For that reason, it took me about a year to understand something that seems so obvious (after knowing it!):

"Ricardo. See this as a form of bodily communication. There is an intention to transmit a message. But you don't understand it. What do you need to understand it?".

The answer was relatively simple! I need to "speak normally". That's it! I need techniques to talk, using the word. In part, I did it with training in coaching and neurolinguistic programming. Later, in Chapter III, I show that this training alerted me to other training needs. It is like this, a kind of cycle that never ends. You study, you find answers, new questions, and a new need for answers and the search for whoever gives them.

THE INTENTION

Intention. This is the word that most aroused my curiosity. Its origin: my course of osteopathy, especially with training in the sacro-cranial therapy. My experience with Susana happened after my first training in "expansion O". Basically, the "expansion O" consisted only in imagining the "energy ball" between the hands. Apparently, the "ball" brought me more than the simple satisfaction of having a "ball of energy" in my hands. Naturally, after the August holidays, when I returned to the course in September, this topic was advertised by me to all colleagues and teacher. I wanted to understand the phenomenon. After all, I was taking the course with people from different areas, namely reiki, acupuncture and homeopathy. Did not happen. I didn't have the answers to my curiosity. I did receive the same astonishment and admiration that I had been left with. Well, patience. It was certainly in my mind the statement of my teacher who said, from the beginning: "You can go two years without feeling anything." Fantastic. In my first training experience, that happened to me with Susana!

For this reason, one of the master's theories was wrong. It is possible to feel "immediately".

That raises the question of what is needed to trigger somatic reactions with our touch. Teaching "techniques"? Apparently not. There was little technique. Just a vague concept of "expansion O". The best was yet to come. Sacro-cranial.

Previously, I already gave you an idea of what the sacro-cranial therapy is. It is a therapy that has the purpose of feeling the movement of the cerebrospinal fluid (CSF), in movements of "flexion" and "extension". It presupposes the movement of the liquid along the central nervous system – brain structures and spinal cord. How does the liquid move? The sacro-cranial cycle is understood to be independent of other cycles, such as the cardiac or respiratory cycle, and independent of muscle contraction. So, how does the liquid move? Part of the explanation comes from the movement between the cranial bones and the sacrum. Basically, there is a "tube" that connects the skull to the sacrum. If the sacrum moves in one direction, the skull will have to follow the movement and vice versa. After all, that "tube" works like a rope: pulling on one side, the other side will have to follow the movement. If this does not happen, there will be a rupture in a more fragile area of the tube.

The movement of cranial bones is the most controversial assumption. After all, in medicine, we learn that the skull joints are immobile. At least, that's what the tests on cadavers reveal: there is no movement. The assumption holds that corpses are not "living organisms", so they work differently. Thus, in a (live) human body, there is bone movement in each cranial bone. As for the movement of the sacrum, the controversy does not arise, especially since in conventional medicine, mainly in exercises for pregnant women, pelvic mobilization is contemplated, and reference is made to the movement of the sacrum. Moving from the main assumptions of the sacro-cranial to the role of the therapist: the therapist's mission is to restore the normal rhythm of the sacro-cranial rhythm. There are references to the number of cycles considered normal in a healthy person, although there is no consensus in the existing literature. Are there common points? Yes. The fact that a low sacro-cranial rhythm is said to indicate, for example, a depressed person and a high sacro-cranial rhythm is, for example, a hyperactive person with attention deficit. The therapist has the role of feeling the sacro-cranial rhythm, placing the hands in specific areas of the body: head, shoulder girdle, solar plexus, hips, thighs, legs and feet. In my "ideal", the head is the starting point of choice (see illustration 9).

Putting your hands on certain body areas has a specific name: *listening*. It is not *listening* related to hearing, but rather it refers to touch: feeling movements of flexion and sacro-cranial extension, respectively of body "opening" and "closing". *Listening* is a term of fascial therapy and not so much of the sacro-cranial therapy. Along the body, we are supposed to feel these movements and, if we don't feel them, we consider that there is a blockage. It is up to the therapist to "unblock", encouraging the body to resume the supposed normal movement. At this point, in training, I admit that I was curious. "How do I encourage the body to resume normal movement?". The answer does not seem to be easy to give, especially if you put a few more questions on the table:

1. Does the person have no sacro-cranial rhythm?
2. I am the one who doesn't feel the sacro-cranial rhythm, but does the person have it?
3. I feel other things than the sacro-cranial rhythm.

Throughout my sacro-cranial training, I have always researched the topic, in books and scientific magazines, and quickly discovered that the evidence on the existence of a sacro-cranial rhythm is practically non-existent. I am not arguing that it does not exist. I am just realizing that there is no evidence to demonstrate its existence. I am not surprised that this happens, especially when almost all existing massage studies report that the effects are purely "psychological". What is missing is to contextualize what is meant by "psychological". Returning to practice: how do I correct the sacro-cranial rhythm, if I don't even know if it really exists? If so, how do I know that it is "what" I am supposed to feel? In addition to these questions, comes the concept of "encouraging the body" to correct. Especially, if I focus on the skull, the sacro-cranial theory states that each of the bones has specific movements and that I, as a therapist, must feel them, analyse deviations from normality and "encourage them" to move in a normal way. Calm! "How do I do that?". The answer to my question is as simple as possible: "With the intention.". Hence the name of this section of the book.

What is the "intention"? The intention is exactly what the name seems to indicate. With my hands still, in a specific area of the body, I will "imagine", "direct my thought", "direct my attention" to the movement I am feeling and indicate the correct way of functioning. Taking the example of the frontal bone, we know from the sacro-cranial theory that it moves naturally in the anteroposterior direction. Naturally, if you feel that this bone moves in a different direction, for example, in rotation, my mission is to transmit the information of the correct movement. Basically, a thought like this: "Frontal bone, don't do the rotational movement and correct yourself for an anteroposterior movement.".

(Break)

I admit that, for a while, I was focused on the sacro-cranial theory, reading, comparing perspectives and asking questions. It took me a while – two months maybe? – questioning the following:

> *If with "intention" I can influence bone movements, what will happen if I have "intention" to go further? To communicate – literally – with my thoughts? What is going to happen?*

What happened exceeded my expectations and I began to have a deep sense of my ignorance in the face of human existence. With touch and with my thinking, I literally started to "speak" to people's bodies. I started to get physical responses to what I asked of them.

Which led me to new questions: "What is the physical body?"; "With what, or with whom, am I communicating?". Does the answer seem easy? It is not for me. At this point, it is necessary to mention the following: for all the cases that I consider to be successful, I have had many others of failure. I grew up and continue to grow with both. When I "fail," it is because there are variables that I am not aware of and that I need to understand. When I have "success", I have it for two reasons:

1. Replication of techniques used in previous sessions.
2. Random factors, in which I work to find "patterns" that will allow me to replicate in future sessions.

In short, it is a work of trial and error, as the theoretical bases are null or practically non-existent and the practice by other professionals does not prove to be convergent with the results I obtain with my own "theories" and "therapy". In Chapter III, I will try to explain the assumptions that guided my practice, the doubts that have arisen, and which continue to arise, and I will identify questions to which I have not yet an answer. However, it is worth mentioning three important points of my "findings":

1. The difference between the conscious and the "non-conscious" is quite evident, during the therapeutic sessions.
2. There is great variability in the way you communicate with the "non-conscious".
3. Communicating with the "non-conscious" is not related to the person's will, i.e., a person who wants to access "latent" information in himself/herself, is not exactly the person who will have results. On the other hand, from practice, many people who showed themselves to be left-brained, rational, and "scientific" had exuberant somatic reactions, beyond their control.

Regardless of how I explain the therapy to the person who comes to me, there will always be an impact on their values and beliefs. Taking the example of Portugal, the Catholic influence is very strong. If we consider that there are sessions where people lose control of their body, while remaining aware of everything around, the association with the concepts of "spirit possession", "exorcism" and "past lives" is very fast. I will try to explain my point of view from these perspectives, in Chapter III. Optionally, I will present you with some of the cases that have marked me most over the past eleven years. I leave aside similar, or less "intense" cases, which I have come to regard as common and transversal to many of us. In all these cases, there is a final learning, important to understand my "logic" of therapeutic approach. In Chapter III, I will present some of the sources I used to deal with the unknown and leave some considerations on everything I learned, especially regarding the idea that we have of health and illness. It is natural that, when presenting these cases, you will encounter some difficulty in understanding where certain concepts or approaches come from. I will try to contextualize them throughout the text, so that I can explain them further in the next chapter.

CASE STUDIES

For ethical reasons, I changed the names of the people I followed. Since 2008, most of these people have been family members, friends, as well as co-workers, former students and their families, friends and acquaintances. I must admit that, until today, I have not dedicated myself professionally to this therapy. There are several reasons for this:

1. I don't have a name to give it!
2. I feel that there is still no "theory" that I can confidently replicate.
3. I have my scientific side to conflict with my intuitive side.
4. Fear of criticism from third parties, especially professional colleagues (totally focused on empiricism and that not even imagine studying something that may seem unscientific. Qualitative methodology is also part of science!). On this last point, with this book, I free myself from my "demons" and I perform a catharsis.
5. Most people want to pay for an appointment and have immediate answers to their anxieties, pains, doubts and other life problems. I don't work that way. I can help to find ways, but I don't say which ones to follow.

Going back to what my father says to me:

"There are as many therapies as there are therapists.".

I created my own therapeutic approach, based on many theories and models. I still can't "fit" it in a specific area. I can simply call it "energetic osteopathy" or something similar. The name would always fall short of its potential. In words, it will always be limited to describe the therapeutic sessions. Ideally, it would be necessary for me to do what I do best: to demonstrate and guide each person, so that they can achieve the same (or better), always considering their background, value system, beliefs and limits. What I present to you is teachable. It is not just for "Enlightened". I bring you cases in which I will certainly touch on "wounds" and controversial concepts.

SUSANA, TRAUMATIC BIRTH

I begin with the experience that marked the beginning of a long period of discovery and exploration. I have already talked about this case, but I will continue it. Susana was the first person in which I trained the "expansion O" exercise. A few seconds after placing my hands on her chest, the body contraction placed her in positions very similar to tetanic contractions. The image that I have the most is that of the head and the tension in the neck (illustration 1). Head in extreme extension and neck looking like it was going to break. More: extremely prominent and throbbing veins. I confess that I was intrigued by those physical manifestations. I must admit. Intrigued is not the right word. Scared is a more appropriate word. I didn't expect anything like that. "What happened here?", I thought.

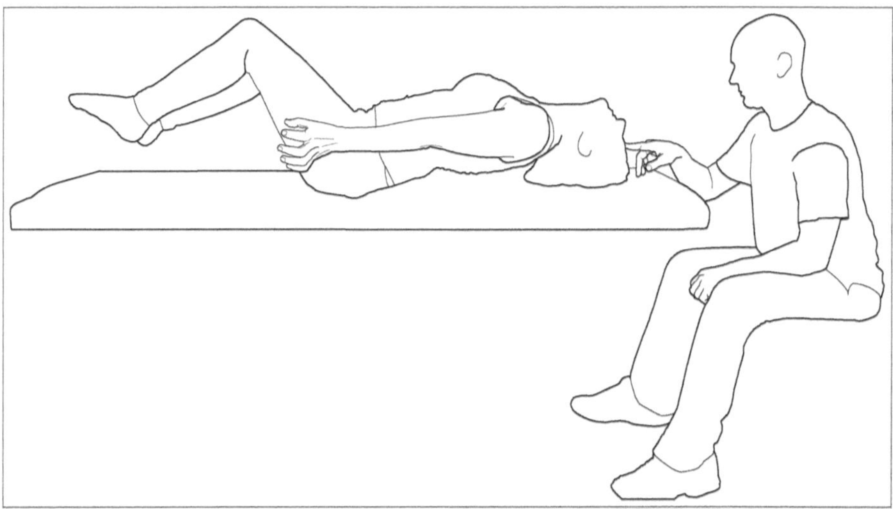

Illustration 1 – In the case of Susana, the following were evident: the extreme extension of the head, the contraction of the upper limbs and the hands "clawed", the arched trunk in the dorsal region and the contracted lower limbs.

Many theories emerged immediately, to justify what I saw. Mythical-religious thinking came first, but it was quickly attenuated by philosophical and scientific thinking. Was it a "demonic possession"? If so, how to stop it? Was it a kind of alien – as in the "Alien" films – that was about to leave the woman's body? It's just that her whole body moved. Literally, chaotic movements were seen from all body areas, especially in the abdomen. Here, it seemed that certain areas were rising, while others were descending, one to one side, others to the other, forming asymmetric elevations and depressions. Accompanying this scenario, we had a groan that was more like anger than pain or other discomfort. The first session passed. Others followed.

Naturally, I had to continue to learn with Susana. The scare had passed, and I was determined to learn a little more. Still afraid, it is true. Fear of the unknown. The second and third sessions were not very different from the first. The same reactions. One difference: I was used to visualizing them. I was calmer and focused on other details. I continued to accomplish what I had learned from "expansion O" – after all, I didn't know anything else until then – throughout the sessions. One thing was obvious. Susana's body continued with uncontrollable physical reactions, but in a less exuberant way. Except for one area: the abdomen. That zone never remained calm. It was as if there was a "being" inside the body, which was contorting anarchically. So, there was light at the end of the tunnel! Body movements focused only on the abdomen. So, what to do with this information? At that time, I was reading some sacro-cranial books and, when reading the author's reports (Upledger), I had some ideas. Basically, I translate these ideas in a very succinct way:

Each cell in the body is independent and communicates with each other. It is possible to communicate with these cells. There are "emotional cysts".

First point. The idea that each cell communicates with each other is interesting. At the age of 28, I started to have a vision of the human body as being made up of "parts". By independent "parts" that communicate with each other. As a health professional and with some professional experience, it never occurred to me to think of the body in that way. Of course, when reading this, there are things that seem obvious: all anatomical, physiological and biochemical relationships take place between different "parts" of the body. It is normal. We are like this. The interesting thing about this case is that my main learning (and which helped me to continue as far as I am today) was based on interpretations different from those that the author had written. An "optimistic" interpretation of the texts read gave me the idea that each cell "speaks" to the next, leading me to question the potential of such discovery.

Second point. If my interpretation had been optimistic, the idea that came to me was obvious and equally optimistic. "If we have cells that communicate with each other, then… why not communicate with these cells?". The truth is that I arrived at these interpretations based on the author's description of his therapeutic sessions. I admit that they were sources of misunderstandings and varied interpretations (as this book will be), but the truth is that it helped me to "think outside the box" – such a popular expression in entrepreneurship and management and, at the same time, so empty of content. The author stated that he communicated with the person's body, but never explained how he did it. Was it by words? By touch? How did he get the answers?

Third point. In the body, there are "energy cysts". Good! Seems interesting! The idea of an "emotional cyst" is like that of a "physical" cyst, only that, instead of containing liquid or semi-liquid matter, it contains emotions. Basically, in a very easy to understand it, it is as if the body accumulated emotions were in the shape of a ball, in certain body areas. Based on this idea, other study opportunities have opened, such as the study of symbolism and body language and, mainly, the study of Gestalt therapy and hypnosis. It is very curious how many therapies say the same, but in completely different ways. The idea of "energy cysts" does not vary much from the concept of "parts" that is also used in psychology and psychotherapy. "Parts". It is something that I will talk about in Chapter III.

Now returning to Susana, I recall that most of the movements were in the abdomen. So, with the concepts I just mentioned, it seemed obvious that there were emotional cysts in that area. Nowadays, I no longer talk so much about emotional cysts, but about "parts". It is a more "neutral" concept, which causes less amazement for people who hear the term. In this case, there were "parts" of Susana who wanted to express themselves. If you were in my situation, would you say that the "part" or "parts" that wanted to communicate with me were...? I won't know what answer you gave to my question, but I realized one thing at that moment. Just seeing the body movements, I soon realized something. Over time, I would have to improve the way of communicating with the "parts". In that sense, I started to study hypnosis, coaching, neurolinguistic programming and to read about psychotherapy. Many theories, many approaches, but all with common branches and similar ideas. Some more "scientific", others more "esoteric", but believe me when I tell you that the similarity between them is great. Carl Jung was also a person who has influenced my work ever since. Interestingly, in Portugal, he is an author that is little valued, or little understood, or else strategically ignored for his ideas "out of the box".

I can tell you that I didn't know which "parts" would be expressing themselves and trying to communicate. But it just occurred to me to ask the following: "Susana, how was your birth?". Most people do not know how their birth went, but Susana knew that, in her case, there had been problems. I don't know what problems, because I didn't keep records of the sessions. It would have been a "normal" delivery but using forceps and vacuum and would have been associated with some cerebral anoxia. Can I translate any "lessons" from this case to you? No! It was my first case, which opened doors for me to continue exploring a wide range of topics and to find instruments that would allow me to communicate with the person and with the "parts" that were manifesting through body movements.

SUSANA'S COLLEAGUES

As I said, Susana was my student and, in the classroom, there were more students. To put it into context, at this stage, I was still perplexed by the results I was getting with the "touch". I was still starting a new phase of learning and experiencing things for which I had no preparation. At least, at the level of formal education. Basically, the massage was an area where I felt like "fish in water", but this kind of result with the touch surpassed anything I imagined. It seemed as simple as "touching" and imagining a result.

Following this work, with Susana, I highlight two more experiences, still within that group: with Elisa and Nuno. Elisa, as a case that was registered as unfinished. Nuno, as an example that the therapy I am talking about is not related to the amount of information learned over the years. It depends on something that, for now, I will refrain from classifying.

I start with the case of Elisa. Elisa is an interesting case. A woman in her twenties, with non-specific phobias, but who expressed herself in a very specific way: in classes, she always had to stay by an open door. Open. Always open. She was full of fears, especially afraid to relate to others. She always maintained a considerable safety distance with others. Curiously, she was one of the first to want me to touch her, after seeing what had happened to Susana. Her curiosity was counter-intuitive, as she rarely liked to expose herself. I may not remember many more details, but one thing I do remember. She smiled and said to me, "I don't believe in this." I smiled. Just as I smile today when people say the same thing to me. What is "this"? I usually tease people by saying: "This what? Exorcism?". For those with training in neurolinguistic programming, this provocation will be the most like the *chunking-down* technique so that, in omissions and generalizations, we can obtain more concrete information. In this case of Elisa, I did not comment. I smiled.

She lay down, I put my index finger in the zone of convergence between the frontal bone and the parietal bones. My smile quickly disappeared. To my surprise, the reaction was immediate. I still believed that there was a large conscious component controlling the movements. Now, if Elisa didn't believe it, she probably wouldn't get any reactions. Pure deception. At the time, and possibly even today, it was the quickest reaction I had to touch. With one finger. Why did I stop smiling? Easy to explain. As soon as I touched her, her face changed, and her colour went from pink to white. She just babbled: "Cold... very cold!". From there, just that. Cold. And colder. Nothing else. The body started to shake intensely and to shiver as if it was inside an ice cube. "Come on Ricardo... seriously? Stop it, because it is starting to scare", I thought. What is certain is that I was unable to find a way to understand what was going on. It just occurred to me to appeal to my training in health and to appeal to a return to consciousness: "Elisa, Elisa, do you hear me? Hear my voice.". Well, she heard my voice, but she just answered "Cold, very cold!". Me and her colleagues put more clothes on top of her body. The body was cold, white and she just trembled. I got scared. There is no doubt about it. But, if things were already unfolding, they had to be resolved. In this sense, I urged her to focus on my voice and the room and the surrounding noise. At that time, I did not know, but this is a technique of hypnosis and returning to the "present". It did not work. The body seemed to tremble even more. If I asked you what you would do in my situation, what would your procedure be? Suggestions are welcome!

Well, at the time, in the absence of help, I really had to use my voice and the "return to the present" commands, so that Elisa could talk to me again. The body was still shaking, but at least she was already talking to me. I asked how she felt. Her description was simplistic. She felt inside a cave and it was cold. At great cost, I managed to bring her to the "present". She started to be more awake for my voice and the presence of her colleagues, but less than expected. The body was still shaking, and it was still white. Visibly, she was not well, and it took a few minutes to get up. The walk. Well, this one was a little bit affected. She was out of balance easily. Some colleagues volunteered to accompany her home to make sure everything was fine. Points to remember: "Ricardo. What happened here?". There was no answer at that time. I still don't have it, currently. I did not continue the sessions with Elisa. Not until I realized more about what triggered the somatic reactions (physical reactions, visible). This session helped my world to start to "fall apart", but it also helped to open new horizons for other areas of knowledge. I am laughing now, because I remembered an expression:

There are people with such an open mind that their brains run away.

To some extent, the expression suits the situation. Faced with phenomena that I did not understand, I could interpret in different ways, but it was important to keep my feet on the ground and to appeal to my critical sense to go deeper into the subject. An obvious obstacle: I had to read more, talk more with different people, I had to get a comprehensive view on the subject, I also had to experience more and more. This case marked me for its radicalism. With Susana, it had been quite scary to see her neck almost break. With Elisa, it was frightening to see and feel the body freezing, turning white, shaking uncontrollably and with the visible "distress" it caused Elisa, her colleagues and me. With what I know now, it is important to retain something: the body can react in the most radical ways you can imagine. You can even go into apnea (without breathing) for minutes. The person may even resemble the dead. I know one thing now: they are somatizations (physical reactions, which want to express something) and do not endanger life. I now advance another learning:

The "body" or the "spirit" or the "soul", or whatever you want to call it, is usually a good "part" and does not hurt either you or the other. It's their expressions that may need some follow-up.

What does this mean? I will detail a little more throughout the sessions that I will describe below. In the case of Susana's colleague, Nuno, I only have positive things to say. It was with Nuno that I was able to evolve. A good "guinea pig" and a good apprentice. With him, I learned that whatever I was doing, it could be teachable. Teachable very quickly! This contradicted what I had learned from my osteopathy teacher who constantly said: "You can be two years or more without feeling anything." (Referring to movements of the sacro-cranial therapy). "Bullshit"! In my first session, I saw, heard and felt more than I ever thought possible. With Nuno, I learned that what I was doing could be taught and learned very quickly. When did I start teaching Nuno? When one of the classmates had a sprained ankle.

Sprained ankle. Until then, as a health professional and with knowledge of massage and osteopathy, a sprain would be treated in a "holistic" way (a very fashionable word that also says so little to those who hear it). This "holistic" form would be the "traditional" form: rest, ice, immobilization, compression, elevation, electrotherapy, stretching and other related interventions. But no. I didn't do it that way. I did it in the "new" way: with the "power of the mind", with the "power of the intention", whatever that may be. But would I do it? No. I would complicate things. I would have a student doing it. Nuno volunteered. From that moment on, and for about four years, Nuno was my "right hand", with whom I learned and tested new therapeutic approaches. With nineteen years old, Nuno was the perfect example for me to "create shock" in the mentalities of "doctors". He got results that left anyone open-mouthed.

So, let's start at the beginning! I just said to Nuno: "You put your hands here and there (on the leg of the colleague who had the sprain) and talk with her foot and ask it to self-treat.". When writing this, I imagine what the reader may be thinking. Ricardo is crazy, esoteric or whatever. I have also been called an exorcist or to have "powers from Beyond". Nothing like that. Let's go down to the earth. In the absence of an explanation of the phenomena, we must find strategies to understand them. At least, I "think" like that. There are those who limit themselves to accepting that there is a "gift" and that it simply "is", and we must live it. I confess that even today I have difficulty "accepting" this way of thinking and being in life. Moving on. There was the woman lying on the massage table, Nuno, and a sprained ankle.

General astonishment, when the woman's foot started to move by itself. At first, with smooth movements that, over time, became more exuberant. Clearly, the foot moved in every possible way and in a very specific way. In words, it is difficult to explain specific movements. For those who understand a little more about the anatomy and physiology of movement, they know that the foot has supination and pronation movements, but that it does not exist *per se*. There are associated with both flexion and extension. In this case, it is as if the foot managed to create the supination and pronation movements in isolation, exclusively, between the Chopart and Lisfranc joints. Amazing! I've never seen anything like it. Nuno looked at me in awe, but curiously without great amazement. I smiled and just said, "Good! To be continued!". The movements there continued and after a short time there was a huge "pop" in the foot. The movement passed. The existing edema was noticeably less. The girl was able to walk again, and without pain. Learning of this situation:

Ricardo, forget what you learned about health and injuries and about your role as a therapist. There is "something" more intelligent and capable of self-healing. As therapists, we are just "there, in that moment", assisting in a healing process.

The most critical may say (as I have heard so many times):

"So, this works for everything?".

Of course not. Let's be honest. There is **no single** therapy that is a solution to all ills. Suddenly, this reminds me of the classes I had on administration and management, in the academic year of the PhD in Administration Sciences, and the "craze" of creating *one model fits all* throughout history. Clearly in the political and economic area and, of course, with the resulting damage. The same will be to say that I do not agree with the vision with which I work daily in hospitals: that the professionals know a lot, they know everything, they are the prescribers and the maximum sages and then... of course... it is made to pretend that cases have been solved and they continue unsolved. I was vague in what I said. On purpose. Anyone who knows the health field will know what I mean.

Let's be pragmatic. Someone has a fracture. Is it possible to heal with the "power of intention"? Not that I know of, no. Infections? It depends! Antibiotics are important. Appendicitis? Well, the appendix must be removed. Don't go there with the "thought". Or maybe it will. Do not know. I have yet to meet the person who does what I hear that exists, but I never saw it: mediumistic surgeries. I believe they exist, but I won't be able to rely on them until I see them. Excuse me. I'm like St. Thomas. I need to see it to believe it. Or to experience. Catholicism's "Bless are those who believe without seeing" is interesting and I even understand its scope. On an earthlier plane, I must disagree. I need empiricism!

The more we focus on a therapeutic form, the more specialized we will become, but the more we will lose the comprehensive view. The more resources we have at our disposal, the more complete we will be. In health, we are increasingly specialized. We do a lot, but of only one thing. We lost track of who the person is and, to fill this, we created the concept of a bio-psycho-socio-cultural-spiritual individual. To say that we are more than the physical, while in practice we remain purely physical. Has anyone ever remembered going to the hospital for "love pain"? No? You should. See/hear/feel the answer you will get. I laugh when people say: "This is psychological!". In scientific articles, "psychological" is used as an easy escape from what cannot be explained.

Moving on...

SOFIA, MY EX-LIBRIS

Sofia is the most perfect example of what can exist regarding the power of touch and the power of the mind (or whatever you want to call it). With Sofia, the reactions to the "touch" took place... at two meters away (because I couldn't get farther)!

To put it in context, this session with Sofia was held at a congress on manual therapies and alternative therapies, which took place in Lisbon, Portugal, in 2009. If I'm not mistaken, it was in the afternoon. During the morning, there had been an interest in the work I was doing, because, as a result of a coincidence, I had "recovered" a person to which someone has already asked the emergency. Yes. As a nurse I decided. I talked to the emergency line and took responsibility from there. The reason? Because I barely put my hand on the back of this lady, who was losing consciousness, and it was as if it was "sucked" towards her chest. Clearly, for me, it was an area for me to intervene. But not in the traditional way and with all health protocols. It took courage (and stupidity) to do so. I did it. Everything went well. Very well!

I will take this opportunity to say this: we must be aware that not all therapies work for every situation. There is no such thing as *one model fits all* or *one size fits all*. We need to analyse the contexts, potentials and limitations of each situation and each person. I remember a potentially dangerous approach that happened in a hospital with a health professional "obsessed" with reiki. A patient went into cardiac arrest and she was found performing reiki. Stop! This is not solved with reiki! You need the life support protocol and drugs and defibrillation. Even if the cause of the cardiac arrest may have been "emotional" (which exists!), it must be reversed in more drastic ways. We have only a five-minute window to act. Solving emotional problems presupposes that the person is alive and has time to resolve outstanding issues (emotional, traumatic or otherwise). The heart has stopped. We must act, quickly! Not with reiki.

Going back to Sofia's case. There I was in the lobby of the congress, talking to other professionals: physiotherapists, nurses, massage therapists and others. In the middle of the conversation and some explanations I was giving, a lady (maybe forty years old) came up with her daughter. She asked me to see her. It is the kind of situations that I am only now beginning to deal with some confidence. Have you noticed that most people ask for help for the "others"? It is here that it becomes useful to study Carl Jung's "Shadow Archetype". Due to projection phenomena, the "other" is the one who always has the problem. This mother had no concrete reason for me to see her daughter. Of course, if someone asks for help for something, it is because "something" exists. I couldn't understand the reason and, as much as I wanted to talk to the mother more than to the daughter (after all, the mother had asked for help), I acceded to her request. With a massage table in front of me, with about ten to fifteen people around me (mostly health professionals and alternative medicine therapists), I asked the girl to lie down. In 2009, I still had no training in hypnosis or neurolinguistic programming (useful for learning some "techniques" of communication). Interestingly, everything I did in that session was a perfect hypnosis protocol. To this day, I think that no script has come out so perfect.

Sofia was lying down. Several people were around me. I started talking to her. Nothing new. She didn't complain about anything. I don't know if this happens to you, but it took me maybe six years to deal reasonably well with the fact that people come to me with "nothing in particular". Searching for "nothing in concrete" is the same thing as the Cheshire cat episode from the movie "Alice in Wonderland" (from 1951):

*"Would you tell me, please, which way I ought to go from here?",
asked Alice.*

*"That depends a good deal on where you want to get to.", said
the cat.*

"I don't much care where…", said Alice.

"Then it doesn't matter which way you go.", said the cat.

Starting a "therapeutic session" without knowing where we are going, gives us room to go anywhere. Obtaining "zero" results can also be a reality. Those looking for "nothing" get "nothing". In this case, I don't know what Sofia won, but I know what the professionals who were there won: a learning for life. I was also included.

Sofia was a seven-year-old girl, with whom I started to speak in a "normal" way. Somewhere in the conversation, it occurred to me to ask what she liked, in order to create an imaginary scenario that she liked and where she could be. Now I know that this is called "creating a safe place" (there will be other names) in regression and hypnosis techniques. Sofia was more than creative! Everything flowed naturally. While she described her scenario, I put my hand on her abdomen, trying to feel any body movements of "parts" that wanted to communicate with me. There were no movements. Sofia was creative, but also suspicious (typical of her age). She always kept her eyes open and in control of the environment. Her scenery was interesting and, perhaps, a pleasure to many: a "super" colourful place, like a rainbow, everywhere. In the sky, on the grass, on the benches. Colour. A colourful, cheerful, "super" setting, where she felt good playing. If I'm not mistaken, there were also colourful candies, scattered everywhere, and swings to fly.

While describing her scenario to me, I asked her to close her eyes. A few minutes later, I started to feel body movements. My hand was all over the abdomen, but the movements came from one area in particular: the area of the stomach and the liver. For those who already have more experience in symbolism and emotions, you will know that these areas are the focus of anger and the source of frustration (the "digestion" of everyday situations). Without almost realizing it, Sofia stopped talking to me. With her eyes closed, the body started to "speak", to move. To give you an idea, this "little exercise" took about twenty minutes. "Things" do not appear suddenly or out of the blue. It can happen, but it is uncommon. The defences are more than many and it is only in cases that I call "pressure cooker" that we have immediate reactions.

So, the scenario was interesting. There was a seven-year-old girl lying on the massage table, I was on her left side, with my left hand on her stomach, the mother behind me, slightly on my right side. In front of me and around the massage table about ten to fifteen people (more appeared, as the session continued). Sofia was lying, with her head turned to the right, that is, to the side opposite to where I was, with her eyes closed. I started to feel the movements as extremely "connected" to me, which led me to do something that I had never done: I removed my hand and continued to "feel", but at two meters away. You know what? I continued to feel her movements in my hand, as if I were touching her physically. The connection was so great that I decided to do a "test". I rotated my right hand (which was in the air, at two meters away) to the right side. Sofia's body twisted in the same direction as my hand. In other words, her body performed a lateral flexion, at the level of the stomach, which forced the entire body to move on the massage table (illustration 2). Surprise! "What if I do it the other way?", I thought. I rotated my hand to the left. Sofia's body spun in the same direction. This time, with flexion on the right side, at the level of the liver. In this position, I felt the stomach area a lot. It was as if my hand were a magnet and the stomach area was a metallic piece. As if pulling a rope, I pulled my hand further away and Sofia's body came dragged. On the part of those who watched, it was intuitive to take an immediate leap to prevent Sofia from falling off the massage table.

Let us stop here.

I don't know what Sofia's "problem" was. I can only imagine. But, unintentionally, I had achieved a greater purpose. I put doubts in the minds of those who were present, and such was the impact that, even today, I remember the words of one of the physiotherapists that was there:

"Okay. I'm surrendered. I always imagined that there could be a conscious component on the part of a person and that the person manipulated or pretended the movements. But with a child, with her head turned towards me and not towards you, with her eyes closed... I can't find an explanation...".

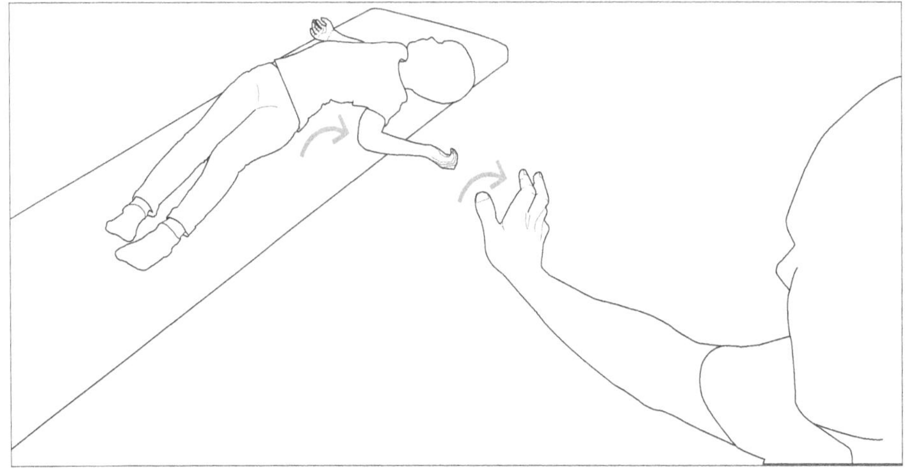

Illustration 2 – Sofia rotated her body, synchronized with my hand. This synchronization took place at two and three meters away. Her head was turned away from where I was.

Me neither, dear physiotherapist. The only difference is that I knew there was something there that needed more practice and more questioning. Above all, to understand what "the hell" I was doing. One thing seemed certain. I knew something that I was not aware of. I knew, without knowing that I knew. Even today, I face this problem. With each therapeutic session, the questions that arose were so many that they started to hinder me and, later, became unbearable. Which culminated in a deep existential crisis, starting in 2011. Only now I begin to "see some light at the end of the tunnel" (nine years later).

Sofia, thank you for your teachings and for your innocence and for having helped other therapists to question human health and existence.

"Distance" treatments like what happened with Sofia are not exactly common. If I'm not mistaken, only half a dozen more people did the same. But it wasn't at two meters distance. It was maybe at eight meters and just because the room didn't allow me to go any further. I have had cases where, without touching the person, the body performed everything my hand did in the air. For example, with my hand over a person's abdomen, if I raised my hand, the body would rise with it. If I put my hand down, it is as if the person was punched in the abdomen. All of it "went down towards the massage table". There also happened to be movements at a distance, only created with my thinking.

Dear reader. I don't know about your experience, but I'm sure of one thing. I was never taught that this was possible. I never thought anything like that could happen. I never thought to do it. My idea of human health had changed dramatically. You may think it is a blessing, or a curse, or the fruit of a troubled mind or some mental illness. You can even think it as quackery, as I also heard.

Whatever it is, if it was rare for me to give justifications for something, then now it was giving me a certain pleasure not to respond to "provocations". I knew I had found something and would have to deal with the criticism that came with it. What worried me the most (and still worries me) were my own doubts and self-criticism. I hadn't found enough explanations for what I was doing.

PREGNANCY AND CHILDBIRTH

Changing a little bit, we go to my experience in the area of obstetrics and treatment by touch and "intention". Still in the phase of discovering a new form of communication with the body, I had the unique opportunity to hold sessions with the mother of my children. From now on I will call her "mother". In this case, during the pregnancy of my first child, during the year 2009. Why do I say unique opportunity? Well, because in almost all the literature you read (be it scientific, pseudoscience, esoteric or alternative medicine) all the advice is in the sense of: "Watch out! She is pregnant!". Well. It is a reality. Several are the factors that affect the pregnant woman. Most therapists do not risk treatment (in any way), for fear of being guilty of something that happens to the foetus. In my case, I would do a treatment with a notion of risk and assuming what came of it. In fact, as I had learned in the last two years, however exuberant they may be, "physical manifestations" would never endanger the life of the mother or the foetus. I remember that my first intervention was in the sense of "educating" my first child. One day, he decided to give his mother abdominal pain. So far it looks normal. The pain was in the stomach area. Possibly, it would be the head embedded in the thoracic grid, on the left side, which caused a lot of pain. As the "mother" responded well to touch (in the sense I have been showing throughout the book), I put my hand on her (already large) belly. I just imagined this: "Afonso, please go down. You are hurting your mother.". Well! I would like the reader to see the movement of the abdomen. It was as if there was an uproar inside. What is certain is that, after five minutes, the situation was resolved. The belly had moved lower and jumped when the head was no longer attached. So far, this seems simple. And for the experience I had at the time, yes. It was simple. It was just saying to my son: "Get down! You are hurting the mother.".

From then on, I thought I could help with pregnancy, in a much more participatory way. If, in fact, I had so much "connection" with touch and with the "parts" of the body, then... let's continue. One of the biggest problems in pregnancy is hip pain. The joints of the pelvis must expand and cause pain. Mobilizing the hip is a Herculean task for any therapist. The possibility of pelvic movements is immense and most of them are almost impossible to create consciously or with the help of another person. So, what did I remember? We will mobilize the iliac and the sacrum. In different directions. With touch and with the "intention" and power of thought. It worked, of course. For the first time, I saw movements that I had never imagined possible. Imagine each of the iliac rotating in the opposite direction. It is as if they "twisted" at the level of the pubic symphysis. This movement was easily seen, especially in the anterosuperior iliac crests. Twisting? Yes. With a difference of 5cm, or more. Believe me. Seeing is the only way to be surprised. Written, it seems easy. It is not. Well, but if it is possible to "twist", then it is possible to move them away and bring them closer together as a way of giving more "elasticity" to the pubic symphysis. No sooner said than done. This also happened.

The hip moved away very clearly. It also squeezed in a notorious way. With this, believe that the pain of pregnancy has decreased considerably. I look at this as pelvic stretches, without those Kegel exercises.

I take the opportunity to talk about pregnancy to introduce another very controversial topic: childbirth. Normal birth? Childbirth with epidural? Caesarean delivery? Let's see. They are all good. They are all bad. It will always depend on the perspective with which we evaluate a case. If the woman has no opening for the child's passage or if the child shows signs of life impairment, then caesarean may be an alternative. In a delivery in which the woman does not control the pain, however many techniques may be used, I admit that the epidural is good. A woman who controls pain, with no apparent foetal distress? Why not normal delivery without any epidural? I will do an aside to talk about the experience of the births of my two children. I will touch on sensitive matters. I already know that when we talk about children, we all become deaf and only channel ourselves into "mine", "it is mine and I know what is best for him" and "I know it because I'm his mother". Naturally. So, even though I know that I touch a sensitive subject, I will continue to give my opinion (based on the experience I have had throughout private practice and based on theories of trauma, sacro-cranial therapy and even symbolism and Spiritism). "Ouch! Now I'm really going to close the book. Enough!", many will say. Yes, close it. Let my foolishness take its natural course. On the other hand, if you are one of those readers that remains close by, I will continue.

Natural childbirth is "natural". La Palice's law applies here. Is obvious. There is no medication. There is no caesarean section. Whether it is possible in all cases? No. If it is encouraged by health professionals? No. At least in my country, especially in the private sector, which continues to encourage caesarean section. We don't need to have a lot of training in business administration and management to understand the reasons behind these decisions. But we cannot just "blame" the private sector. In the public sector, the use of epidural is overly encouraged and there are even some paradoxical situations that I still cannot understand. To explain them, I will use the experience of my two children. Before doing so, I would just like to leave a compliment to the mother of my children who, although our relationship has ended, I continue to see her as a great woman. At least, in the sense of childbirth.

The anxiety of the birth of the first child is enormous. Who is already a parent will know it. Who is not, will learn when they go through this situation. The mucous plug was released on January 5, 2010, around 11am. We knew it would be a matter of hours before our first child was born. We chose to wait for the development of events. For now, there were no major contractions. We both agreed that the delivery would be normal, without an epidural. Most female readers must think: "Who are you to think and decide for the woman?". I clarify we were both in agreement. The father's role is essential during the childbirth process to maintain the partner's peace. If you want any more help to convince you (in case you are a woman, of course) it is the fact that, in the preparation sessions for childbirth, both parents are present. Right? Because it's important! It is important, but apparently forgotten on the day of childbirth, as I would later see. The day went by without much news, even though we knew that, at any moment, we might have to go to maternity. This happened around 2am. Arrival at the maternity, consultation with the obstetrician and decision to intern in order to start childbirth process. So far, nothing new. I accompanied the "mother", carrying the kit of clothes, hygiene and the baby's first change and entered a corridor. A professional colleague was at the door of one of the offices. Visibly tired, as is typical of my profession, she uttered a phrase that, even today, I remember vividly: "The pains you have now are nothing. In a little while you will see what will hurt you!".

What?

Obviously, I would need an epidural myself if someone told me that! They teach us that pain is subjective. We have scales of different types to evaluate it, but it remains subjective. The "mother" was in pain, but she endured it. Something similar would happen at the birth of my daughter. We then went up a floor, they told us a place to put most of the clothes on and we went into a delivery room after a few minutes. As it was at night, apparently everything was calm, except for a woman who was nearby, screaming, in pain. Not a great encouragement for anyone who intends to have a normal birth. Meanwhile, I found that the husbands, or companions, of the women who were in the delivery rooms, were absent. They were the same men who were in the reception room when we arrived at the maternity, almost two hours before. The women were screaming. The men were drinking coffee and talking. Very good. Men! Support your women, especially at this time! Pain can be controlled with support, with words of encouragement and affection. Remember that, please. In the meantime, we entered the delivery room. Perhaps it was 4am. My son was born at 12:22. So it was a long waiting. In between, we had the visit and monitoring of an anaesthesiologist and two nurses. They were very concerned because they did not expect the delivery to be performed without an epidural. "To the full force", they wanted to prescribe and administer the epidural. Bad luck, or "coincidence", the "mother" had platelets too low and, therefore, they gave up. What I want to call attention to is that the professionals never considered the hypothesis of not administering an epidural, although that was the clear intention on our part. Well, apparently, there was also no one who was minimally prepared, or interested, in accompanying the delivery, with all those breathing exercises that are learned in the preparation for childbirth classes. That is why I say that men are essential. I spent almost ten hours replicating all the exercises I had learned, focusing on her so she could hear me (Yes. Labour pains make the woman "deaf"). Very interesting, was the fact that a cardiotocograph was available to see when the next contractions would be. There I saw some numbers going up and I already knew that the contraction would be "more" or "less" intense. Every time the medical and nurse staff opened the door of the delivery room, the values of the contractions skyrocketed and the "mother" lost control. I thought: "Wait Ricardo, this will be resolved!". With the shift change, at eight o'clock, for my happiness, a nurse came in with very good sense. She was already aware of the situation (not having taken the epidural) and was smooth throughout her communication approach. Which gave me the confidence to ask her who would be needed to deliver the baby. She told me that only she would be needed and that she would call a paediatrician after birth. Wise words. One of the problems in my profession is that people (in general) do not give us due value or recognition, which makes us somewhat defensive and powerless. In this case, I just told her: "You have all our confidence. Please close the door. We don't want interruptions.". So it was. Despite being the first delivery and there was much pain, controlled with breathing exercises, my son was born without any problems, with more than 4kg!

In my daughter's case, we've had similar cases as well. Especially from a colleague of mine speaking loud and clear: "Oh, you don't want an epidural? Is the husband who tells you not to take it?

Husbands here don't have a word. I don't want to hear shouting and crying in here.".

What?

I have no words to describe. For the first time, I had to be a little hard and affirm our position. It is not surprising that three nurses passed by us in an hour. Until the most experienced nurse came on and offered to help with breathing exercises. Within two hours of entering the delivery room, my daughter was born, safe and sound. Once again, we had given the nurse full authority to perform the delivery without the presence of other professionals. In this case, neither the paediatrician was needed. I also remember two nursing students, from the Maternal and Obstetric Health specialization, who looked at us and just commented: "it was the fastest delivery we have seen. And the first without an epidural!".

First, I want to clarify that this is far from being a "boastful" attitude on my part. What I am telling you has a meaning, which I will explain to you. Before the birth of my two children, I already had the necessary knowledge to understand that, in order to avoid future problems in their evolution, they would have to be born "naturally". In sessions that I had had until then and already with knowledge of regression therapy, I started to detect that a large part of the physical manifestations that people presented were related to birth. The problems I had already seen alternated between:

1. The period before conception.
2. The period between conception and delivery.
3. The postpartum period.

If you are a fan of past lives and reincarnation, now is the time to get excited!

How did I get access to the information that was provided to me by a person's own body? How did certain information become "conscious"? From a period prior to the conception itself? That is, at a time when, possibly, the parents had no idea that they were going to have a child? Amazing! Or even the information obtained from the period before delivery and after delivery. Some of the reports I heard were impressive, as they were so clear and objective. People present at the time of delivery, problems that occurred, conflicts between family members, and much more. Of course, my scientific background does not allow me to plunge "blindly" into any theory that easily explains or tries to explain a phenomenon.

It is true that I studied exorcism (in Chapter III, I dedicate myself to talk more about it), but also other theoretical perspectives that recognize that "past memories" can come from genetics, from mitochondrial memory, from the very sensory memories "of this life". Or other "lives". Very interesting is the Gestalt theory and the immense work developed by Carl Jung, so that we can analyse these phenomena in another light. But beware! I am not saying that reincarnation does not exist and that we are not the fruit of some energy that is out there on the loose. Nothing like that. I keep that possibility open. The advancement of science begins to get closer and closer to proving the subtle "energy exchanges" between people and the environment. Jung already said that! Eastern and Western philosophy too! Many others! I remember an anecdote from a teacher who tells his students that oxygen had been discovered in the 18th century. One of the students immediately asks: "Teacher, so how did we live until that date?". Oxygen was always present. But it was not "seen". The same will happen with these things of "energy", "collective unconscious" and "past lives", "disease transfers" and other things. However, we also must question and use common sense to assess whether these subjects are not used by people just to get attention (very common). I talked to some psychologists to have their interpretation of the sessions I was conducting. For most, schizophrenia and schizoid personality were very desirable labels.

From an early age, I began to realize that the therapeutic sessions were posing a big problem. On the one hand, there were therapeutic sessions that nobody could explain to me, or even replicate. Sessions that culminated in "cures", not resolved by other traditional routes. Some of the sessions looked like authentic exorcism sessions. People squirming and making movements that would never happen consciously. In many sessions, I found myself talking to specific areas of the body, talking with diseases, among other "parts". A myriad of things that have shaken my belief system and made me more fragile. More fragile, for having recognized my ignorance and for feeling the "weight" and the need to study an infinite number of areas, to understand certain phenomena. I was interested in analysing different perspectives and therapeutic approaches. In the end, many of them say the same thing, but in different ways. The issue of birth is one of the areas in which I have devoted some study.

What is birth? What represents? From the perspective of Spiritism, birth represents an unhappy moment. Contrary to what most of our society thinks: being born is life and life is joy. For Spiritism, this only means that there is a "being", a "spirit", an "energy" that returns to this world (already from itself inferior) to learn new lessons not learned in a previous life. I like the idea of Spiritism as a way of looking at life, but I cannot forget other ways of thinking and questioning life. From an osteopathic and trauma perspective, I realized that the moment of delivery is unique. If we add the theory of Spiritism and even theories about "birth" and "rebirth" throughout life (some psychological theories focus on the symbolism of rebirth throughout our life) we get an interesting perspective. Being born is a trauma. Let's see. The baby must cross an extremely narrow channel. For this, it has its own instinctive biomechanics, which allows it to exit without problems. For example, one of the shoulders retracts and the cranial bones float to let the head pass. Being born by natural childbirth is the same as saying:

"I overcame my first obstacle and I didn't die!".

On the other hand, according to the sacro-cranial and osteopathic theory, cranial movements at birth will give what I will call "the rhythm of life". If you imagine a motorcycle, it is the same as that "kick start" movement. It is giving the energy for the engine to start. It is to give the child the opportunity to "enter a life", with confidence that he or she has overcome a possible death.

Born with epidural. Childbirth is not natural, in the sense that most contractions disappear. Contractions are the baby's "kick start". It is the contractions that wake up and prepare the baby for the difficulties of a new life and for the potential threat that is in front of him or her: going through the birth canal. Many of the women have perfect labour. With pain, that's for sure. Many of them when they are about to give birth and have an epidural, lose their contractions and the baby no longer seems to want to be born. Many end up in caesarean section. Let's face it: this happens frequently. On the one hand, fortunately. This way I will have more and more clients to solve problems related to an "unnatural" birth. I am often asked this question:

"Ricardo, what problems does a non-normal birth bring? Caesarean or epidural?".

"Concretely", I admit that I don't know. But I know the most common problems that arise in connection with this. Disorientation in life, insecurity, pain in different body areas (neck is common), diseases resulting from emotional somatization, bodies to position themselves "automatically" in foetal positions and to perform rotations typical of normal births. Yes! It's amazing how I could see these movements, in detail, in an adult! It is as if we have an adult model to replicate what is described in obstetrics books. Fortunately, one of these sessions is filmed, from beginning to end. I'll talk about it later.

It is difficult to say what is derived "concretely" or "objectively" from an unnatural birth, as we are the result of multiple variables. However, and this is factual, in most regression sessions or sessions in which I "speak" with bodily "parts", I am referred to the time of birth: umbilical cords around the neck, people at birth who should not be present, babies who are removed from their mothers at birth, parents who did not want to be parents, envy of people close to their parents and others.

Imagine what it is like to be born by caesarean section. Imagine that you are at home, inside your bed, on a cold day. In your home, and in your bed, you are feeling warm and protected. Now imagine that a stranger enters your home without your permission. It's bad enough, right? Now imagine what it is like to go to your room, take off the clothes that keep you warm, and throw a bucket of ice all over your body. Do you like the feeling? I would not like it and would become aggressive if I could defend myself. Well then. The baby cannot defend itself and this is the feeling that is transmitted to him/her. Someone opens the mother's belly, goes there to pull it with their hands (the outside temperature is not the same as the temperature of the mother's womb!), many times you have to "undock" it and force it to come "out here". The baby does not defend itself on the spot but will do so in adulthood when he/she has the opportunity. The memory of such a birth is recorded and will be activated in the future. As in the case of Susana, who had her body movement centred in the lower abdomen, for issues that would be related to her own birth.

It is unpredictable to know how and where the memories of our existence will be stored. Possibly, in the case of Susana, the somatizations were related to birth and to the relationship she had with her parents (I could not develop more at the time, nor did I have the knowledge I now have on the subject). Memories can be lodged in the ovaries and uterus (in the reproductive system) and can lead to the (physical) appearance of irregular menstrual cycles, amenorrhea, the appearance of benign or malignant tumours and other things. To a certain extent, it is a memory that "traps the whole system" so that the person cannot reproduce and so that situations that occurred in the past are not repeated. Or simply, in the case of Susana, she received a memory from her mother and took it as her own (without knowing it and possibly without wanting it). As you can see, there are many interpretations for each case. In most of the sessions, in my country, I would easily have someone who would come out of the office and say that he or she was "afraid of these things", that he/she "respected whatever it was" and that because he/she was an "open address", he/she would go out to not be possessed by a "demon".

The potential of emotions and their somatization is very poorly understood. It is my conclusion. It is not enough to go to the psychiatrist or psychologist. No. More is needed. More capacity for professionals to intervene in fields that are still hidden and face traditional values. In Portugal, we still have Catholicism deeply rooted. On the one hand, it is a source of values, on the other hand it is a limiter to our ability to question. Our political past will also not have helped us to become a "modern people", more intervening.

NUNO, THE REBIRTH AND THE "TWO FACES"

In the continuation of the previous case, I speak to you about Nuno. Talking about this case is easy because it is one of the few cases that I have recorded on video. I don't have many sessions recorded on video because privacy is something to respect. Not everyone accepts to be "guinea pigs" or to expose their lives to a camera. Nuno was a precious help so I could test some theories and approaches. My "connection" with his "non-conscious" was very good, which allowed me to test new therapeutic approaches. What happened in the session I address here, was done with two more people. Two massage therapists, both reiki practitioners. They wanted to understand a little more of what I was trying to explain to them about somatic reactions, as they had never witnessed any (despite working with "energy therapies" for many years). So, there were four of us in a room. Nuno on the massage table, the three of us with our hands on his body, waiting for some somatic reaction. Some muscle contractions started to occur – which was already expected. After a few minutes, the unexpected happened. Nuno began to be in a foetal position (which I see frequently in therapeutic sessions) and to show signs of suffering, on his face. The body seemed to contract with its own rhythm. Sometimes it relaxed, sometimes it contracted a lot (remember what I said about maternal contractions during labour?). At the time, I didn't care. For me, it was just contractions. Different from the ones I had observed to date. They became more intense, which led me to suggest that we put Nuno on the floor. So, we did. It didn't take long before something happened that, on the one hand, scared me and, on the other hand, still makes me laugh today. Nuno's head started to rotate, as if he were in the birth canal. Everything felt like it was coming out of a "birth manual". Surprising was the moment when the head propelled the whole body upwards. I will try to make the image clearer. Nuno was on the floor, lying on his left side. His upper limbs were contracted, as if they were "squeezed" against the trunk. The head was rotating to the left and resting on the ground. Out of nowhere, the body leapt into the air, in an attempt to upright and support itself only on the head. Obviously, such phenomenon did not occur, because the body fell just after this impulse. The head could not bear the weight of the body, especially with such a sudden impulse. I know one thing. Consciously, it is not possible to carry out that movement. Even if that was possible, training worthy of an Olympic athlete was necessary. That was not the case. At that moment, I remembered something I had read about a similar case. The author, Upledger, said that he had used "assistants" to create an improvised birth canal. Hmm! Now I had two more men in the room. Great! One would simulate the birth canal, with its upper limbs forming a circle. My other colleague and I were going to hold Nuno and put him in this "birth canal", for him to be "born". Why not? So, we did (illustration 3). New surprise! We did not facilitate the passage of Nuno. We offered some resistance to its passage. His entire body was lifted into the air and descended through the "channel" until he touched the ground. When his body touched the ground, Nuno just said:

"Wow… Wow… It's like I took a bucket of cold water and as if a wave had caught me and turned me around! Weird!".

Does this remind anything? I can say that, at that moment, such was the amount of novelty and information, I could only concentrate on "this is fascinating". I did not connect to the "cold water bucket". For me, Nuno was dry. Dry! Objectively, he was dry. He felt different. He felt strange. After a couple of days, I watched the footage I had made of this session, to review and analyse it with other "eyes". I still remembered almost every detail and continued to revisit, time and time again, the moment when the body propelled itself in the air to be just supported by the head on the floor. Then, the passage through the "birth canal" and the "I feel wet". Eureka! "Ricardo, how did this escape you? What if this 'wet' is the amniotic fluid?".

Questions:

1. "How are there memories and movements of a normal birth, if Nuno was born by caesarean section?".
2. "Do we already have a code embedded with the entire 'manual of common procedures of the human body'?".

For me, it became obvious that it was limited to rely only on the touch and the resulting somatization. I needed to communicate by words and not just interpret body movements.

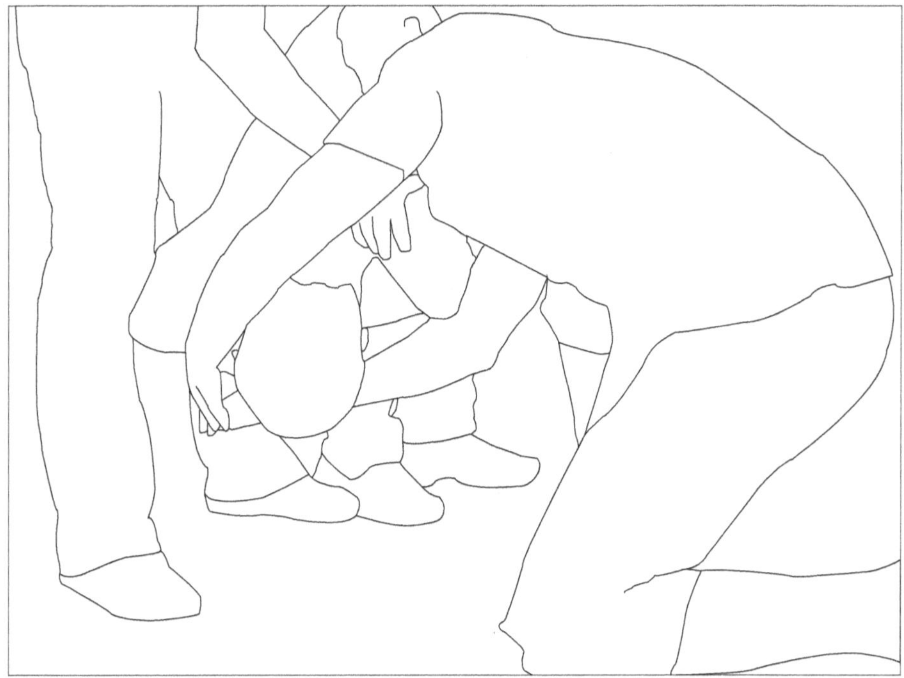

Illustration 3 – Nuno went through an improvised "birth canal" with the help of three people.

Still talking about Nuno, in one of the sessions, a very interesting situation occurred. With my touch, it was common for Nuno to go into a "trance", almost immediately. A trance is understood as a state in which a person is aware of what is going on, but watches phenomena that are beyond his or her conscious control: body movements, emotions and feelings flowing. In this session, which I called "two faces", the involuntary and rapid eye movements were all too evident. Something interesting happened: every time the head rotated to the right (no matter how small the rotation was) Nuno laughed. Laughing out loud. Each time the head turned to the left, Nuno cried. Compulsively. When writing, I get the feeling that "this" is something simple. On the one hand, laughter. On the other hand, crying. The most difficult to understand and experience is the transition from a "hilarious" state to a "sad" state in less than a second. I believe that Nuno was getting tired of these transitions. Even today, I do not understand what was behind this somatization. The "two-sided" reaction was the only time it happened to me, so I include it in this book. If the reader knows how to interpret this reaction, I will be happy to analyse it.

CLÁUDIO AND "MESSAGES FROM BEYOND"

Cláudio's case occurred in late February 2011. From that date on, my life changed radically. Probably, many situations led to this change: children, economic crisis in Portugal and experiences that exceeded my ability to understand. The year 2010 had been rich in intuitive experiences. I had dreams of situations that ended up happening in a short time. I knew where to go, I knew what I wanted, and I had insights into life like never before. In January 2011, I had a dream in which, very clearly, I got the message: "You will have the opportunity you are looking for.". From hearing so much about "spirit guides", I was always curious to go through a situation where I could talk to them (if that exists). There is the "power of intention", the "power of attraction" and these New Age fashion theories. Being sceptical, I have always remained open to experiencing something like that. In January, my dream told me that I was going to have that opportunity. "When?", I thought.

It was faster than I thought: a month and a half later. Cláudio was one of my sacro-cranial students and, in my classes, it was common to learn from real case studies. With each other, but also bringing people outside the course, so that I could guide them in practice.

Cláudio had a back pain at the level of D9, which we never came to understand the meaning of. If I'm not mistaken, the medical diagnosis was spondylitis. Of course, considering the diagnosis, I always looked for the "meaning" that could exist at that level, not just a physical problem. After all, since 2008, it was common to find different origins for problems that manifested physically. Three years later, I came to know that Cláudio was finally beginning to understand the pain, using regression sessions. At the time, I couldn't follow him, as he is from Lisbon and I from Porto: three hundred kilometres away. Apparently, the pain disappeared with the daily intake of açaí berry.

What happened then in this session? In one of my "experiences" of trying spinal pain treatments, I decided to invite all my students to put their hands on his body. We place our hands at the level of D9-D12, both on the abdomen and on the back. The pain seemed to have increased and Cláudio started to change his face. So far, everything seemed very normal and usual. I was used to watching muscle contractions in different parts of the body. But when I looked carefully at an area that I consider "vital" for the therapy that I "created" – looking at the rapid eye movement – I noticed that the face expression was different from anything I had already seen. It did not take many minutes for something that is not common to watch (but that has happened more than once) to occur: the loss of consciousness of the person being touched. It is not too much to repeat some essential points.

What I am talking about in this book is a therapy that "only" consists in touching a person and "hoping" that there will be communication on a "non-conscious" level. It can happen by body movements, by words, by writing. Regardless of the form, one thing is common, and it should be so: the person is aware of everything that happens.

The experiences are to be experienced and reanalysed through various prisms, so that there are moments of problem solving and eventual cure (in the literal sense). Having said that, for me, it is already normal to see the astonishment of a person looking at his or her own arm moving by itself and without being able to control it. This movement is almost always linked to my thinking and my "requests" (both mentally and verbally). Yes. Just imagine and things happen. Without speaking and without influencing the "conscious" person in treatment. What is there in common? It is the existence of the "conscious" and the "non-conscious".

In this session with Cláudio, after a few minutes of touching, by all the students present in the room, the "conscious person was gone". In other words, we couldn't get any answers from Cláudio. It is as if he had suddenly deafened. As if he had lost his touch. Eyes closed. I noticed that the hands started to get tense. Not just the hands. The upper limbs, especially the right. In his right hand, the indicator appeared, and it seemed to be indicating to one of the students. So he stayed a few seconds, until I had to intervene and ask: "Is it related to this student?" Cláudio's mouth half-closed said something like "Yes!". "Is this the best therapist for Cláudio?", I asked. "No!", was the reply. Meanwhile, in my mind, a series of mental protocols, theories emerging, doubts, alternatives for action, assessing what would be going on there and how I could explore the whole situation. It didn't take much to realize what might be happening there. "A voz!" ("the voice", in Portuguese), said Cláudio. We all look at each other. The student who had his finger pointed at him asked if it had to do with the "voice" (his or Cláudio's). "No!", again. "A voz!" (the voice), insisted the "part" who was using Cláudio's mouth as a communication channel. "What voice?", we wondered?

Until I remembered. Calm. It is not "a voz"(the voice)! It's "avós" (grandparents)!

Calm! Was that what I was thinking? Was this a session I hear so much about? Was this a relative already deceased, of this student? I had many theories, but this session shook them all. There were no frames of reference to frame what happened from there. In fact, "Cláudio" called practically all the students and me, in the minutes that followed. A different message to everyone. Deceased relatives transmitted messages to each of them. Something that only made sense to them, because each one cried when they heard certain things. The messages were transmitted almost with the ears of each student glued to Cláudio's mouth. Those who watched, tried to hear what was said, but nothing made sense to us. Only to the listener made sense. It was very evident that it made sense, from the way each one reacted. At that time, Cláudio no longer had his finger pointed. He grabbed people and pulled them close to his mouth so he could speak.

Before all this happened, I still tried to "interpret" the situation in a different way. When the hand pointed at the students, it looked like it had eyes. He knew exactly where each one was. I thought: "Well, but Cláudio had already seen them before going to the massage table.". Now, Cláudio had his eyes closed and pointed to each one. I would have to change the variables. At the most silence, I asked everyone to switch places. We did this about two or three times, with radical changes of places. In all cases, the finger always pointed to the right person, to whom he had to say something.

"Okay, I give up. I don't have interpretations for what is going on. Let yourself go and see what this gives. Just assume that it is an entity external to Cláudio using the body as a channel to communicate with us.", was what was on my mind.

Meanwhile, it was my turn. To date, there are only two or three people to whom I have told what I have been told. Totally symbolic and subjective for those who read or listen. "Guide them to the Light!", was what was said, with a slurred speech. I still remember having my collar choking me, because Cláudio was pulling me hard with his right hand, so that I could hear him. What scared me, I admit. I only imagined images from "Alien" movies or those horror films, with a suspense song. "Would Cláudio take my ear off?", was my deepest fear. I was afraid to let myself get closer. Which made Cláudio pull me even harder.

"Guide them to the Light!", was the message.

It made sense to me, given that most of the past few years had been dedicated to training people in the health field, especially so that they would be open to seeing "existence" as something more than the material plane. But I had a lot of doubts and constantly came up with thoughts: "Ricardo, you can't change everyone. Most do not even want to know anything you have to say to them or try to show them.". Not to mention that, professionally, it would be useless to say something like this: "The disease has a spiritual or emotional origin" or "cancer is in the person to self-destruct the entire system, since the person has not changed standards of living, but is willing to regress under certain conditions". Ufff! It was a lot for me, so this message came at an opportune time to keep me on track of what I consider to be the fate or destiny.

"But everyone is a lot. I can't.", I replied. Then I was pulled hard again, closer to Cláudio's mouth. "All. All. Guide them to the Light! All!". Well, things didn't seem to be famous. All? Ufff... At that time, I already had enough shoulder pain (excessive responsibilities). "Everyone" was something that overwhelmed me even more. Well, but if in fact I was talking to some "spirit guide" or a "non-physical entity", possibly it would be able to take that pain away from me, right? So, let's ask. And I asked. "Well, I already understand that is 'all of them'. But I have a lot of pain in my shoulders. Can you get rid of that pain?". Cláudio dropped my collar, put his hand on my neck and started to give me small knocks. Light but very fast strokes. Very, very fast. You know what? The pain passed. The pain in the neck and shoulder girdle was suddenly gone. I thought: "Go get it Ricardo! You were kidding, but the truth is that now you have been left without answers once more and your questions are and will be more than many.".

Lessons to remember:

1. This session made me question my entire practice and the concept of "existence" even more.

2. Once again, as with Susana in 2008, everything I was taught could be wrong or very incomplete. After all, we still don't know the answer to the old and classic philosophical questions: "Who are we, where did we come from and where are we going". But, perhaps, there are even those who know where they are going. At least it is the message that many scientists send: "You die. There. There's nothing else.".

3. Learning from Cláudio had been very "obvious", but it made the bridge with other previous sessions, with other people, at other times. There were sessions where I suspected that it was an "outside entity" talking to me. But this could be just because there are memories stored in certain areas of the body and not necessarily being a deceased person or a "spirit guide" (see Spiritism, in Chapter III) using a "communication channel" to express oneself.

After this session, I was left with doubts that forced me to return to earth. I went down so much that from 2011 until today, my life has been adrift, without much meaning, without great insights, with painful moments in between. At that moment, I felt that a part of me had died and another part had been born. Death and birth felt so vividly. In a way, in the past nine years, I am relearning how to live. In a completely different way than I had done before. This book marks a moment when I feel ready to spread these experiences, without much fear of the criticisms that have haunted me for years. Not only the criticism, but also the "overvaluation" of what I do. It both drains my energy that person who attacks me to say that the reactions that people show are the result of a previous combination between both (between me and that person), as well as that person who travels to me, sometimes covering hundreds of kilometres, in the hope that I have a crystal ball or that I put my hands and "call me to the Beyond", so that I can talk to Luís Vaz de Camões, Napoleon or Julius Caesar. In the case of reiki practitioners, that I connect myself with the "reptilians" and present to the world the higher teachings that we must follow.

"No.".

We must solve our things on Earth, here in this world. That's what I learned. Regardless of how we do it. Do I believe there are people who see dead people? Yes. Do I believe that there are people who have mediumistic abilities and who help to communicate between different "energy plans"? Yes. That there are people with the capacity for immediate healing, just touching the person? Yes. Do I believe in astrology? Yes. In numerology? Yes. All of this is symbolic, but it works. It gives the same results as a psychological test but put another way. No, I do not see myself in those scientific studies that say that all this is "bullshit". Until today, it has not been possible to prove certain things? Yes. May the evidence say that "complementary and alternative medicines" don't work? Yes. Most of the time, this is because the studies cannot be compared with each other. The other reason is the lack of studies in these areas. Please! Even today, the scientific literature is clear to say that massage does nothing: it does not increase skin temperature, it does not cause effects on muscles, tendons, it does not cause volume changes, and other things. Basically, it is "psychological". Right! The old concept of "psychological" always comes up when we don't know how to explain a phenomenon. But I would like more people to come to this "psychological" and to solve, for example, the pains of emotional origin, without resorting to antidepressants and benzodiazepines. Because it is possible to get there. In ways that are not always "scientific". Did I ever imagine treating headaches in a few minutes, just with the touch of my hands, on a person's head? That my hands in the air would move a person's body, at eight meters distance? If there are any scientists out there who want to carry out studies on this, go ahead! I also want to understand what I do! It is easier, to later teach and replicate.

THE WRITING SHOULDER

The "writing shoulder" is exactly that. That session in which I spoke with the right shoulder of one of my students, but instead of using her mouth to communicate with me, it used a pen and paper. That "part" that identified itself only as "shoulder" and that wrote on the paper "more pressure". The girl was one of my sports massage students. She was finishing her Occupational Therapy course. I considered her a sceptical girl. Her own age and higher education in health helped her to be so. More sceptical. More rational. I remember a dedicated, attentive girl with body pains that she endured intelligently. These pains were centred on the hips and knees.

We always analysed her pains from a biomechanical and physiological perspective. Physically only. Until one day, when at the end of class, she told me she had a pain in her right shoulder. She would probably expect an osteopathic treatment. I chose to place my left hand on her right shoulder and my right hand on her right hand, waiting for some movement of the body that would indicate the "reason" of the pain or that some movement would begin that would lead to the correction of the problem. I confess that I was little confident that she would have any reaction. An apparently rational girl could be an obstacle to treatment of this kind, although my practice told me that this has nothing to do with it. I had seen many people wanting and having high expectations and the result was… "nothing". Others, on the contrary, wanted to prove that "none of this existed", that it was not possible for the body to move outside of voluntary control and… wow! Within seconds, their theories were defrauded.

In the case of this "shoulder", things went well. The right upper limb became tense (very tense) and started to move on its own and just to carry out the movements I mentally asked of it. Curiously, the girl was looking at her arm, she had no control over it, but she still didn't seem overwhelmed. Weird! Well, I continued to "speak mentally" and asked the shoulder to correct itself. Thing that insisted on not happening. The movements simply repeated what was on my mind. If I imagined the hand moving, it moved, the arm going up and there it went. But it did not correct itself. In other words, I was "connected" to a "part" who wanted to talk to me, but who expected something more from me. Self-correction was probably not possible. I asked aloud if the shoulder could use the girl's mouth to speak to me. In vain. I looked like a "silly". Asking the shoulder to talk to me. Where had this been seen before? Meanwhile, other students were watching and there had been about fifteen minutes. For the first time, I remembered something different. "What if it's a pen and paper?", I thought. I asked again, out loud, if I could communicate with the shoulder and have it answered by writing. "Yes", was the answer she gave with her right hand, after a command I had standardized (see ideomotor reflexes, in Chapter III). If the right hand moved, it would be a yes. The left hand, a no. These movements became known as "ideomotor reflexes" or "ideomotor effect", in the 19th century, and were widely criticized by the scientific community. They were and are criticized. What is certain is that, the "suggestion" or whatever you want to call it, made the right hand move and, thus, I promptly gave her a paper and a pen.

For the first time, I watched the "non-conscious" writing.

A rigid upper limb, without writing quality, almost without knowing how to hold the pen. It was like watching my four-year-old son draw or write. For better or worse, there was the following: "More pressure". This phrase came as a result of something that had already begun to manifest. The shoulder moved by itself, but it didn't seem to "get anywhere". Apparently, it needed more pressure. I laid the girl down on a massage table and pulled out her upper limb. Shoulder movements have increased (a lot). It looked like the shoulder was going to come off the trunk. I've never seen so much movement of the shoulder girdle. I take this opportunity to inform you that the shoulder girdle is probably one of the "biomechanical phenomena" in our body. There are several forms of articulation between the shoulder blade, humerus and rib cage. A real challenge for massage therapists, osteopaths, physiotherapists and other professionals. All the joints moved, but it still came to nothing. Seeing this treatment was surreal!

It is as if the "therapist" was just the "employee" of the shoulder, with the shoulder getting irritated and "pointing the finger", as if to say: "It is nothing like that!".

In fact, more was needed. More minutes and more pulls of the upper limb (I admit that I was afraid of a dislocation, such was the strength with which I pulled the upper limb). At a certain point (understand after about twenty minutes!), there was a huge "pop". It was easy to understand. The shoulder had managed to correct the problem. If you ask me where the "problem" was, I don't know. It was in one of the joints, but I don't remember which one. Anyway, it didn't matter. As soon as the shoulder gave this "pop", the movement of the right knee began, with the same intensity of movement.

"What???", I said out loud.

"It cannot be! Now I don't have time to continue the treatment, but I already understood that the hip and knee pains will probably be related to this shoulder pain. Can it stay for another time?", I said aloud. The knee stopped the movement. The girl's body was generally calm. It was an agreement. I could go on, at another time. That time, it didn't happen. The girl didn't look for me anymore. I was sad, I admit. Knowing that I can contribute to a "cure" or treatment that is frankly superior to other forms of treatment, I am saddened when people do not seek it. Lessons to be learned:

1. Either people don't value what I do, or they are afraid, or they don't want to improve themselves. It may be something else that I don't think of now.
2. For each "success" session, you will have a "failure" session. Why do we only count the experiences in which we were "successful"? This is particularly visible now, for example, on social media. We only advertise the good times, the moments of euphoria, the moments to take a *like* and few *posts* to say "I failed". Probably, what we see as failure is what allows us to reach another level of knowledge that improves us.

The reality is that the shoulder pain was gone. There were left only to treat the hip and right knee.

HEALTH FAIR AND THE "RESTLESS HIPS"

May 2009. At this point, everything was new. I had not yet experienced other sessions that went far beyond this one. However, there was a session that marked me intensely. I was at Exponor – the largest congress centre in the north of Portugal – participating in a health fair and giving demonstrations of massage, hot stones, osteopathy and sacro-cranial therapy. There were plenty of interested persons, although there were several companies doing the same. So, I would have to be different. Obvious! The sacro-cranial therapy was going to be my bet. The idea was even attractive. Sitting at the head of a massage table, with my hands still on a person's head and just limiting myself to "imagine" healing and involuntary body movements in response to my thinking. Several people went through me, many of whom were health professionals. With good response to touch and involuntary movements. But nothing that surprised me much. To whom I did it, yes. It was surprising. How did body movements exist when my hands were still?

I know. For the most sceptical the answer is: self-suggestion. Right! I've heard that many times.

Of all the cases I have seen, there is one that stands out. It was the first case in which body movements were associated with a possible malignant tumour in the uterus. I say "possible" because I didn't have contact with this lady anymore, to confirm this fact. For the diagnosis, she needed to perform a biopsy. The outlook was not encouraging. This session is a reference because I have it recorded in *full-HD* and it is easier for me to re-analyse it whenever I want. In fact, it is a reference I use in the training of manual therapy professionals. It was only at the end of the session that the husband informed me that there was a possibility of a malignant tumour, but that they were still waiting for the results of tests. With this information, it was with another interest that I saw and reviewed these videos.

Describing this session in words is not as easy as explaining when viewing a video, but it will still be easier than describing other sessions in which I have no audiovisual record. Therefore, I was at Exponor, in May 2009, with several people around me: her husband, two physiotherapists, trainers and trainees and, of course, spectators (who blocked the entire stand). I was doing a sacro-cranial demonstration (some say that what I do is not sacro-cranial therapy!). A lady appeared, lay down on the table and I, as usual, put myself in the position of choice to assess the subtle movements of the body. That position is to be seated at the head of the massage table, with my hands on the head of the person who is lying down, thus being able to easily visualize his/her whole body.

In this specific case, I paid some attention to the temporal bones, which were the ones that showed more "subtle" movements. In this zone, body movements started immediately. Almost as if my hands were a giant magnet and the lady's body was metal. When touching, the abdomen, chest and head were tense. The head was extended and turned slightly to the left. The face expression looked like pain and suffering. Almost immediately I had a reaction very typical of the "most successful" sessions: my eyes closed tightly, as if I couldn't even open them. In 2009, I thought it would be sleep. I would just be tired and sleepy. The feeling is similar as if I wanted to fall asleep right now. The closing of my eyes was intense, and I couldn't control it. Consciously, I closed them even more in an attempt to open them again. When reviewing the video, to describe what happened in this session, I can't help but smile. My face is like someone who just woke up. It was 3:54 pm, on May 10, 2009. I had already woken up a long time ago and I felt good. Still, I thought it was sleep. Nowadays, I know that it is a sign of the beginning of communication with the "non-conscious" of the people in front of me. In fact, the reaction of people with a "rapid eye movement" (REM) is a strong indicator that I have already established communication with the "parts" (see Chapter III).

It was precisely the REM that started to appear in the lady who was lying on the massage table. If we are more precise, what happened was like REM, adding a strong movement of the eyelids, which were shaking at great speed. A person in REM enters a phase of sleep, in which it is possible to dream. In my case, in most cases, REM is a strong indicator of the likelihood of being able to communicate with the "non-conscious", just with my thinking. With questions and requests. It happened in this specific case. My mind was focused on asking for an increase in somatic manifestations that would help me understand what they meant.

The lady's head began to turn, both to the left and to the right. The movements became so wide that I was forced to get up from the chair and stand up to accompany them. Meanwhile, the lady's hands began to tighten and landed on her abdomen, slightly below her navel. At the same time, the trunk started to "twist". The area of the body responsible for this torsion was the hip, which rotated both upwards and downwards, around a sagittal axis located in the sacrum bone. Naturally, the hip when performing this movement forced the lower limbs and the spine to adapt. So, alternately, we saw one lower limb getting shorter than the other. Obviously, the limbs did not shorten, but the rise in the hip was so great that it seemed so. The abdomen contracted and relaxed, alternately. The tension in the hands remained. The movements did not stop there, because after a few minutes, a new detail was added: the chest began to expand beyond what was normal. Interestingly, it just looked like it was doing it in the anteroposterior (front-back) direction and not in the lateral direction. Which is strange, as this is not common in ventilation mechanism. Suddenly, the hip movement stopped. The hands relaxed. The movements started to focus only on the chest, which stopped expanding and started to move sideways, alternately. It is almost as if you were watching *hip-hop* movements or a Beyoncé dance. The movements were isolated and asymmetrical. It was as if the body was trying to get rid of restrictions. It was as if it wanted to let go of something. The lateral movements stopped, and the chest began to rise and fall. The trunk seemed to have a life of its own and there seemed to be a person in the back pushing the body upwards. Underneath, there was only the massage table. Hip movements and head movements restarted. Keeping my fingers in contact with the lady's head was already a difficult task. The movements were too fast and too wide. Difficult to follow. At this point, I know that I could remove my fingers, because I felt all the movements of the body, very obviously. I just didn't do it because I had a lot of people seeing, who could interpret what I was doing in many ways. I thought, "Let me keep my hands here, because people think it's a new type of massage.". Yes. I heard that comment: "What massage is this?".

The movements were now global, from head to toe. Which didn't last long. A novelty: the scapular waist began to move from top to bottom, which forced the upper limbs to move. Imagine that you have a person on your shoulders, and you make every effort to get him/her off your body. In this case, the movements were similar, but accompanied by violent contractions of the abdomen and deep inspirations. The alternating movements of chest expansion and contraction and abdominal contraction and relaxation were frightening. They were too fast and too wide. The head started to spin violently, from side to side. For the first time, I really had to let go of my hands. Which made me confused, although I was excited by the newness of this session. I still didn't want to pass on the public image of a treatment without a physical touch, so I went back to touching the lady's head with just one finger! As I was smiling and talking to a physical therapist who was at my side, whoever was attending the session did not seem concerned. "Thank goodness!", I thought. For most, "that" was just a new type of massage.

Well, the movements were too strong and wide. I decided to change my strategy: "I will counteract the movements." By thought? No. Physically. It was faster. I then placed myself in front of the person, with my right hand on her abdomen. The movements were almost all linked to an extreme abdominal movement. How extreme? Extreme! It was only now reviewing all the videos of this session that I realized something that I had already forgotten. The abdomen "struggled" with me. How? Imagine a lady in her forties, lying on a massage table. Imagine your hand on her abdomen. Now imagine the abdomen, and just the abdomen, pushing all your body weight up. Yes. The trunk, more precisely the abdominal area, had more strength than any that I could put on it. I spontaneously did what I now call "setting limits and imposing rules" (see Chapter III). "Get down!", I said aloud. Yes, this time it hadn't been by thought. It was a direct command. "Get down!". Simply this. At this stage, I had a lot of excitement around me. It would not be the case for anything else. What? A "Ricardo Vs abdomen"? Interestingly, with my verbal command, the abdomen stopped rising and started to rotate intensely. Violently. So much that I asked a reiki colleague to come and help me. My intention became one: to resist movements, to see what results I would get. In fact, it is a principle of the sacro-cranial therapy: to identify resistances and to counter them. In general, it is a principle that exists in manual therapy. So, I did. Until I lose my strength. Then, together with my colleague, we agreed that it would be time to ask for the session to end. Ask whom? Well, that now leaves me with no answer. It would simply be asking. "I'm going to ask the body," I thought. And it worked. The body started a series of movements in which it normalized on the massage table and relaxed. Completely. As for me, I had no strength in my upper limbs.

The lady was fine. Practically unaware of the movements she had made. When I asked this lady about a disease that could be connected to the abdominal or hip area, the husband informed me of the possibility of a malignant tumour in the uterus. They were waiting for a biopsy. Whether it was cancer or not, I won't know. I learned that:

1. The body has a Herculean force, when moved by non-conscious forces.
2. The energy of a tumour (malignant?) is huge and "gives a fight".

In this session, I just regret not knowing what I know today. But it is normal in our lives. It is the experience. It is trial and error learning. It is personal and professional improvement only possible with practice. With successes and failures.

CRISTINA AND PSYCHOGENEALOGY

Moving away from somatization cases, I present a case of psychogenealogy. What is psychogenealogy? Psychogenealogy is the analysis of your family, down to the details that we can identify. It is to analyse your ancestors. It is to find out the reason they gave you your name. It's finding out what your piece (or role) is, in a familiar puzzle. It is to discover why you act as you act. It's finding your way. It is to discover your mission in life. It is this and much more.

This session was unique. Unique in many ways. Unique because the person left "cured" only with that session. Unique as it was a short session (less than two hours). Unique because it was my first time to do something like that. Like this, few more existed. To solve a problem, which I can consider complicated, just in one session? Rare. Very rare.

I do not remember all the details of this session. I remember the big picture, which is what I'm going to present here. One of the details I don't remember is the lady's age. She was probably about sixty years old. I will give her the name "Cristina". Cristina came to me by a friend's reference. Cristina could not mourn the husband who had died, about a year ago, and lived in permanent suffering and sadness. Outside, her friend said depression. Ah! Depression. So many causes. So many reasons. So many different reactions to that state. "Ricardo, how are you going to approach this problem?", I thought. "By touch?" or "By word?".

Well, I started with touch. The body movements were not as exuberant as I expected, but they allowed me to realize that there was a huge pressure on the chest. Regarding the symbolism of the chest, we have two essential feelings to analyse: the sense of belonging, coming from the heart; grief or deep suffering from the lungs. In Cristina's case, the body reflected, in fact, what was going on in her life: mourning and a sense of belonging. The husband had passed away.

Instinctively, I chose not to continue with the touch. The body had already given me a clue as to the path to healing. It was as if to say: "Ricardo, the problem is here in the chest.".

So, I chose to explore a subject that then aroused my interest and which I was exploring: psychogenealogy and repetition cycles in our lives. Repetition cycles, or repetitive cycles, are not a unique concept of psychogenealogy. The concept also exists in kabbalah and Spiritism.

I then went on to build a Cristina's genogram. Without going too far. I didn't even need to. There was already a repetitive cycle "that jumped in the eyes". At 39, Cristina had lost her father, which had been a very important milestone in her life. Now, at about sixty, she had lost her husband. Again, the cycle of suffering, associated with the father or male figure. The loss of the male symbol. Cristina had a daughter. "How old is your daughter?", I asked, but already anticipating the answer. "39," she replied. I didn't have many interpretations at that moment. I took the repetitive cycle for granted. This lady's daughter was on a repetitive cycle. She was repeating moments of the mother, in this case of the loss of the male symbol. If Cristina did not go beyond this learning or if she learned nothing from this situation, her daughter would most certainly go through these trials. Is this concept of psychogenealogy scary or interesting? We all have our own history and our story.

I chose to take an approach in which I went through Cristina's traumatic moments, only focusing on the male figures: father and husband. It seemed obvious to me that this was an important part of family learning, as her daughter was already in a similar cycle. It had to be broken. With regression techniques, I managed to get Cristina to relax (it was not difficult because the hypnotic trance already existed, due to the "connection" that had been made with touch), created a safe haven and returned until she was 39 years old. Basically, I created a meeting between her and her father. I'm glad I did. The reaction was immediate, and I can still see her raising her arms as if hugging a person and crying.

My intervention consisted of following this process of reunion, so that both "parts" were satisfied. Fortunately, everything went well. Cristina said everything she wanted to her father. The father said everything he wanted to Cristina. It was then time to "let go" of the father. Let's move forward. "Cristina, proceed to the moment immediately before your husband's death.". Once again, the perfect session. Everything was flowing. This time, Cristina was in the "presence" of her husband. As with her father, Cristina embraced an invisible being and cried (not as intensely as with her father, which is not surprising, as the traumatic focus was on her father and the experience with her husband was a reflection or repetition). Both said what remained to be said.

I brought Cristina back to her safe haven and, from there, to the living room and the time where we were. Cristina's face was very, very different. No tension. More pink. She thanked me and hugged me. Later, I learned that her life had changed radically. She had come out of her depressive state and had a different relationship with her daughter and everyone around her. Her life was taking a new turn. I was and I'm happy. It is not common to have a cure with just one treatment.

Fortunately, "miracles" happen!

HEADACHE AND THE RIGHT OVARY

Several times, one of my trainees (whom I will call Liliana) asked me to help her with her headache. Maybe she has asked me half a dozen times, but I always apologized for not seeing her. Sometimes, due to lack of time, other times due to tiredness. Headaches are common to one hundred percent of people. However, its origin can be varied, ranging from a simple imbalance of cerebrospinal fluid circulation (in the perspective of sacro-cranial therapy), to aneurysms, SOL (space-occupying lesions) and much more. In short, anything can cause a headache. It is therefore necessary to conduct a comprehensive collection of information to explore possible origins. In the case of Liliana, the pain had existed for several months. It was a deep, constant pain, as if the head exploded. She was followed by medicine and took medication. It didn't seem to work. She tried other non-pharmacological therapies. Nothing worked.

"Ricardo, can you help me with my headache?", she asked me once again, at the end of one of our classes.

I smiled and said yes. After all, it would be the seventh time she asked me. I asked her to lie down on the massage table and, once again, I sat down at the head of the table and put my hands on her head. After a couple of minutes, I still felt nothing. No movements.

I waited a little longer, but without high expectations. After a few seconds of my "early withdrawal", I started to feel body movements, but only focused on the head. Liliana felt them too. The movements were not wide. They were short, of little expression. The headache intensified over time, but there was nothing to show me the way to treatment. Just movements and pain in the head. Until the moment when she screamed and brought her right hand to the abdominal area. More precisely below the navel and just on the right side. The pain was notoriously localized. The fingers of her hand pressed against that area. "Liliana, the headache?". The headache was gone. Just like that. From one moment to the next.

"Okay, Ricardo. The headache is just a reflex zone. The problem comes from that abdominal area.", I thought. If this case had happened in 2009 or 2010, it would be a case like many that I had had: a lot of somatization and little understanding of its meaning. This case occurred in 2015, so I used other resources that I had at my disposal, namely using the "word" to talk to that abdominal area. Hypnosis was not necessary. Communication with a body "part" was already done. I just had to ask that part to agree to use Liliana's mouth to talk to me. Does it seem strange to you? I understand that it can be.

This technique does not always work. Sometimes, as was the case of the "writing shoulder," the form of communication must be done through writing. There are other forms of communication, as I will speak in one of the following cases. In the case of Liliana, the abdominal area gave me a signal that it would be possible to communicate through speech. That area did it after I parameterized "I cannot answer/ I don't know/ you are not allowed to explore". Usually, I parameterize that involuntary movements on the right side will be a "yes" and that involuntary movements on the left side will be a "no". In general, the movements are visible in the extremities (hands and feet), but I have seen them in the eyes, knees and other areas. Read about ideomotor reflexes in Chapter III.

I then went to the abdominal area and simply asked the name it wanted to give me. No response. It is usual for the "parts" not to identify themselves. In fact, the name is a too small word to describe something that can be much more complex. Let's look at the example of the word "God" and the meaning it can have from person to person. In the absence of a name, and seeing Liliana's abdominal area, I chose to ask directly: "Is it the right ovary?". "Yes!", was the reply. Still, I continued to screen for other locations: intestine, liver, gallbladder, bladder, uterus, among others. "No.", was the answer to all of them. Thus, I had a precise location, which is not always possible to obtain in all sessions. It makes subsequent work much easier. "Ovary, how can I help you?". This question is not always successful, but it is the one I like to use because it is direct, and the answer requires a "superior wisdom". It is as if the body has an "internal doctor" who knows the origin of everything and the form of healing.

In this case, the ovary asked me for something that makes me smile even today: heat. "Heat?", I asked it. In my mind, the thought was: "Heat? Just heat? Seriously?". The answer was also simple: "Yes.".

It was not difficult to realize that the desired heat was not from any infrared lamp or paraffin or other type of equipment. It was the warmth of my hand. Liliana's pain was gone at this stage. I put my hand in the area where Liliana had hers and asked the ovary to let me know when it had all the heat it needed. So it was. At the end of ten minutes, Liliana said: "It's done. Thanks!". It seems simple.

This simplicity can heal. What did I do in these ten minutes? I just talked to Liliana. Nothing specific. Just a trivial conversation, until she felt the need to tell me: "It's done. Thanks!".

That case reminded me of another one I had in the past. The case of a girl who appeared to me with similar pains, but not so focused. A girl with a lot of personal problems. At the time, my approach had been to touch and follow the somatization that was taking place. This session was not particularly different from many others, except that it was one of those that have scared me a lot. Four hours after being with me, she urgently entered the hospital and was diagnosed with appendicitis. She was operated and looked good.

I must tell you that I was not the one who gave her an infection of this kind. In fact, even if I said it out loud, no one would believe it. If it was in the Middle Ages, the most that could happen was me to end up at a fire for witchcraft. No. My interpretation of this case is more in the sense that there were repressed memories in that organ and, in the impossibility of being removed in another way, the choice was to be removed by surgery. My touch only has accelerated this process of emotional release, so that it immediately came up and became visible to everyone. As far as I know, after this surgery the girl has improved considerably from her personal problems. More I can't say. In this case, I am in doubt if I could have avoided this surgery, if I already had experience with hypnosis and if I used the "power of the word".

The lesson to be learned is that it is possible to accelerate somatization by touch and trance.

Based on this experience, I suggested that Liliana consult a doctor immediately, in case of symptoms such as extreme pain in the region or signs of bleeding (signs of a problem in the uterus or ovaries). I was convinced that that session had only served to make the ovary to manifest. It could not be in my competence to continue this treatment. What has been confirmed. Two weeks later, after several tests at Liliana's request, a tumour was discovered in her right ovary. I didn't have the courage to ask her more. My job was done. I had just been a vehicle that had decoders to "hear" that Liliana's body zone. The problem then became visible for others to to find it and to solve it. Two years being followed by doctors and none had found the cause of the headache (initially it had been a diffuse pain in the abdomen). In just an hour, the cause was discovered. Fortunately, Liliana is one of those people who does not conform to the answers they give her and was open with her doctors when saying that "someone" had told her that there would be a problem in the right ovary. Answer obtained: "Do you still believe in these things?". I smile and wonder what "things" are those that everyone refers to. Mythical-religious thinking in action or just an inflexibility of thought and action created by scientific thinking? Science is necessary. Let it be clear what I say. Science is necessary. However, it gives no answer to everything that a human seeks and everything that does not fit in the "box" is classified as "artefact".

ANA, A RIGHT KNEE AND A LED LAMP

What relationship is there between Ana's right knee and an LED lamp? Probably nothing. Pure coincidence. But I had never seen an LED lamp releasing smoke (intensely). In this case, the phenomenon occurred at the very moment when I asked for the presence of Ana's father, who had already passed away. Strange and scary! But it may have been a coincidence. Let's talk about it by steps.

It was a summer night, in 2015. Ana and two other friends were at my house and we were talking about various subjects. Somewhere in the conversation and connecting with the dozens of books that are on my shelves, the focus of discussion centred on the topics of health, body and linguistics and the way they all relate. Excited, I was sharing my experience and giving some examples. It wasn't long before I was ready to demonstrate some of my theories. I just can't seem to be quiet and talking. I must do things. So, what did I choose to demonstrate? I performed some tests that are adapted from applied kinesiology (see Chapter III). I then used muscle tests to get answers from the "non-conscious", through parameterization done *a priori* in my mind. In this case, I used the upper limbs to perform a simple "yes" and "no" test (see the ideomotor reflexes in Chapter III).

I asked several questions, in the face of some amazement from Ana and her friends. All the answers to my questions were right. I was interested in exploring more, and so I started asking more and more questions. I already knew that there was pain, especially below the hip. Specifically, on the knees. Both? Yes. On any special? Yes. In the right. Now, I already had the experience to know that the right side refers to the parental figure (not necessarily the father) or the future. So, I started to have some more specific indicators of the source of the problem. Attention! Ana could have physical problems in her knees! Usually, I am not just looking for physical causes. I look for other causes. I usually say that the physical body is easy to treat, but this will only be possible if we understand why injuries, illnesses or accidents may be occurring and affecting certain areas of the body. In Ana's case, the pain was located on the right side, which, symbolically, is related to the parental or male figure or future. I've read books that say the opposite. That the right side is feminine. I don't agree with that view. My whole practice shows the opposite. The symbolism is constant, whether in body language, in the analysis of writing, drawing or even religion. Returning to the right knee. The knee represents flexibility. Why do you kneel at Mass? Have you thought about it in a symbolic perspective? Mass is symbolism. From beginning to the end. Religious symbolism is not my forte, although I recognize that it is quite enriching to understand body symbolism. The knee is, therefore, a representation of our hardness towards life. Left knee pain? Problems related to the maternal or female figure, such as the mother, a sister or a female friend. It may also be related to a past problem or related to both: a past problem, originating in a female figure. Pain in the left knee may indicate that the person has difficulty dealing with past problems. It can also indicate that the person has an enormous desire to "walk in life", but that he or she may be doing it too fast. Right knee? The opposite: paternal or male figure and temporal relationship with the future. Pain can indicate that the person has difficulties in "moving forward with life", for fear of encountering obstacles or not feeling prepared to act.

In Ana's case, I started to explore her relationship with her father and brothers. Apparently, all right. Nothing bad. As I am stubborn and I know that what people tell me is, in most cases, an omission or misrepresentation of reality, I prefer to trust the signals given by the body. There was a problem with a father figure or prospects. Of that I was certain. In this specific case, it was not necessary to use *chunking-down techniques* (exploring a subject thoroughly), as Ana's knee took on a life of its own and started to shake. To her amazement, her lower limb was out of her conscious control and was now "connected" to me. From here, I knew that everything would be easier. It is more gratifying to communicate with the "non-conscious" than with the conscious (limited to several levels!).

Ana was so scared that she started to apologize. After all, her relationship with her father was not good. It was a distant relationship and one that became more distant because he had passed away a year ago. "After all, I was right!", I thought. Despite being happy to get this detail right, something worried me. Ana offered a lot of resistance to any question that related to her father (there are many reasons for this to happen. One of the most serious? Sexual violence. Not that it was the case.). Her body responded to all my requests. If I thought the body would stop, the body would stop. If I asked it to move, the body would move. I then chose to use *perceptual positioning techniques* (although the name may vary), common in psychodrama and constellations. My idea was to join Ana with her father, similarly to what I had done with Cristina (see previous case) and her father and husband. Ana resisted this proposal, but, still, it was my intention to request the "presence of the father".

At this point, one of the LED lamps in my living room began to emit strange noises, as if it were "clicking". I didn't give it too much attention. I was focused on what I was going to do next. Spontaneously, I asked Ana's father to introduce himself in the room to talk to me (it is a technique of perceptual positions!). It was then that Ana's friends called me and pointed to the LED lamp.

"Ricardo, is that normal?". The 5W LED lamp was releasing smoke heavily. The light went out, but the smoke was growing all the time. It forced me to stop, to fetch a ladder, to look sideways at one of the extinguishers I have at home (just in case), to go up to the lamp and remove it.

It may have been a coincidence. It may have been more than that. The session ended there. I realized that the relationship between

Ana and her father was a subject that had "too much energy" and that it would be better to wait for other opportunities.

THIS IS NOT THE WAY YOU WILL COMMUNICATE

Following the previous case, but not in 2015 but in 2010, there are similar points with the case that I will tell. I was in a sacro-cranial therapy course, as a trainer. For me, trainees should be trained in practice. Theory yes, but they must practice. If not, how can I guide them? All trainees could take people outside the course, so that we could use them as case studies and, of course, be our "guinea pigs". In this case that I present to you, the guest came from my side. He was a colleague of mine, perhaps ten years older, from the NLP Master (Neurolinguistic Programming Master) course. I got along very well with him, although I was always "provoking" him, because he was in a repetitive cycle, which he couldn't get out of. Extremely rational and inflexible, he was unable to analyse the relationship with his daughter and his deceased wife. Something blocked any attempts to address the issue. He consciously spoke about them, but his words did not convey emotion. Not because it was "cold", as you might think. I felt there was something else there. So, I invited him to attend one of our classes. In this session, I just chose to let all the trainees get together to analyse the life of this colleague of mine. To some extent, I was waiting for new insights into the case. The conversation with him became interesting, going through moments of provocation and tension. Still, my colleague was cordial in how to counter the provocations. He was also studying neurolinguistic programming and communication techniques. These techniques are useful for many areas from psychotherapy, to marketing, to "brainwashing", hypnosis and more. Therefore, caution is needed with its use and a full awareness of its impact. The truth is that we never know what the impact will be.

To soften the atmosphere, I suggested to my colleague to lie down on a massage table that we had right in the middle of the room. All those present were seated around this massage table. I then asked them to use touch to "listen" to the body. I don't remember the details, but I know that more than two trainees evaluated him. Two of them achieved results. With one of the trainees, the body had become tense in the abdominal and thoracic region. With another trainee, who I will call Rosa, well, the reaction was unprecedented: she started to swell her belly (yes, it was very visible) and to eructate. I had read about such cases when I studied Spiritism (see Chapter III). Eructation was a sign of communication with spirits. The truth is that I had never witnessed such a phenomenon. Until that moment. I suggested that Rosa sit down again and leave the rest of the session to a classmate. So it was. I don't quite remember the details of what followed. However, I remember that we reached a stage where my colleague just had thoughts about his dead wife. "Great!", I thought. It would be a way of seeing to what extent these memories had been stored in the body. My colleague visibly struggled with emotions. It was notorious. It was as if he did not want to release them and, rational as he was, he was getting confused because he was losing control over them. It was then that things escaped my predictions. As I looked around the room, I noticed that Rosa was changing her face. What was changing so fast? I can't explain it in words. It was a very special change. The skin changed colour, the micro-expressions changed radically, the breathing changed, and the eyes rolled. It was as if I was seeing a mixture of epileptic seizures with the first signs of a stroke. Scary, yes, and no one had noticed yet.

I remember looking quickly at my colleague, on the massage table, at the current somatization, and looking at Rosa. There was a synchronization of movements!

Instinctively, and very quickly, I got up from the chair, ran over to Rosa, put my hands on her head and it just occurred to me to say out loud and firm: "Rosa, stay focused on my voice and on my touch. Stay focused on my voice and on my touch. Focus on the voice!". Then I continued:

"To whom is trying to communicate, I have to say that this is not the way. It's not the moment. Not without asking Rosa for permission. Not without asking permission from those present in this room. This is not how we will communicate. Is there anything to say? Already understood. We all understand. But we will do it in another way, at another time. If you understand what I am saying and if you accept it, I ask you to return complete control to Rosa.".

It was immediate. Rosa returned to her usual face expressions, but visibly tired. As for me, I just remember to keep my hands on her head and stare at her. Dry. Determined. That moment transcended everything I had ever experienced, but I was happy to have been able to deal with the situation.

I had had similar cases before, but I always saw the somatization in the person I was treating. It could be a memory that was stored. It could be an area of the body that needed help. I had never seen "something" communicating by someone else. For me, one thing is obvious. Just as I do not like people entering my home without authorization or invitation, I do not accept intrusions of this kind.

It was an instinctive reaction. It was a reaction that only had as a background the acceptance that we are more than what we touch, that there can be energy transfer and that this energy may even be intelligent. A linguistic "trick" to say that I would be treating the matter as if, in fact, my colleague's wife was communicating with the physical world, through a channel (Rosa). Got it. It was present. But, for that, I needed Rosa to be aware of these characteristics and to know how to deal with something similar. Which was not the case. So, I hold on to that conviction. Communicating yes, but with respect and permission from both sides. Do you see any similarity between this case and the manifestation in an LED lamp (see previous case)?

MENTAL POP-UPS

We live in a digital age and all of our devices have applications with pop-ups, whether these are windows that open to remind us that we have a scheduled meeting or advertising that opens without authorization for us to buy the latest model of any smartphone. The case I present to you is the same as a pop-up, but in this case a mental pop-up. In the cases that I have presented so far, I said that there are several ways to communicate with a person's "non-conscious". Sometimes by touch, sometimes by word, sometimes by writing, sometimes by a mixture of means. In this case, I present another form of communication: through the mental path.

The case took place with a long-time friend, and we have only recently talked about this issue. For some reason, I felt I had to include him in this book. I was still in my initial exploration phase of my "new" manual skills and being sensitive to communicate with each person's "non-conscious". This friend of mine was showing signs of depression and, therefore, I asked him to serve as my "guinea pig". Why not? Everything would be learning. Well then. In fact, I was able to have immediate somatic reactions, but very confusing to me. His whole body was twisting, and his jaw was clenched intensely. It felt like accumulated anger. The whole body trembled and moaned. As I was still in the exploration phase, I went through several areas of the body, to realize which would be the area that would most react to the touch. This area was in the liver region. It is not surprising, as the liver is linked to anger. On the same plane, there is the stomach, which symbolizes the ability we have to digest day-to-day life, its experiences and the way we deal with frustration and our actions. Actions that are not always consistent with our will and our intuition. Thus, internal inconsistencies appear, between what we know would be a good path and the actions we have to keep to stay adapted to the world and to the expectations of family, friends and co-workers (see Chapter III, subchapter of "body language").

Therefore, I had one of my hands on the liver area, with my friend's body always twisting intensely. The clenching of the jaw and the moans were aggressive. Would he hit me? I did not know. I had never had anyone with such aggression in front of me. I didn't know what to look for. I didn't know how to get out of that situation. At this stage of my learning, I was just alert and sensitized to improve touch. However, in my mind, I was always asking for something that would help me understand. Then, suddenly, the shape of a person came into my mind. Faceless. Just a figure, with feminine shapes. The colour of the hair and its shapes appeared to me. Blond hair, just below the shoulder, slightly wavy. I thought it was a strange thing. What purpose had that image? Was it the product of my imagination? Was my mind creating something just to make my ego calm and satisfied? What is certain is that the image never left my head. It was intense. There was no more information. Just that shape. As I had nothing to lose, I just said to my friend: "Look, I don't know the origin of these bodily movements, but the image of a woman, blond, with wavy hair over her shoulder appeared. I don't know if that makes sense to you.". I ended that session there. He just smiled and told me he knew what it was. This may have been in 2008 or 2009. Only in 2016, we returned to this issue. It had remained in our memory. Finally, after seven years, I had the answer to my doubts. He showed me a picture of an ex-girlfriend. The figure fit that passport photo perfectly. He asked me: "Was this girl?". "Yes! That's right!", I replied. The puzzle was complete. The breakup had been traumatic. He was unable to "digest" the situation and was still angry (liver) for things that had happened. From learning it remains that, in the absence of communication through touch, word or writing, we can still count on communication via mental pop-up.

PAIN IN THE LEGS AND THE BURDEN LEGACY IN CHILDHOOD

There are strange things. As I said at the beginning of the chapter, most of the people I saw were outside the main profession, as a nurse. I did not publicize (and still do not do) my therapeutic approach because I did not know what to name it and because I was still afraid that people would seek me out looking for miracles. I cannot promise results, despite the many successful therapeutic sessions I have had. This case is strange because I got a call from a lady who wanted to try a session with me. Honestly, I don't know how she got to me. Not for advertising, not for ads. On someone's recommendation? Perhaps. What is certain is that she appeared in my centre. Smiling. "So, what brings you here?", I asked her. "I don't know!", she replied. Well! If there are answers that made me confused (they still do) it was when someone was looking for help but didn't know why. It reminds me of that moment in the 1951 film Alice in Wonderland, which I spoke of in the case of Sofia. Someone who seeks help without knowing the way to go, must be prepared for everything that may come to him or her.

After exploring the reasons that could have led her to look for me, something more objective was identified there. This lady, whom I will call Andreia, was 39 years old and had a pain in her left shoulder for some time. Interestingly, nothing specific. She didn't know how long it had been there or how it had come. Apparently, she was not even confused with that pain. The perfect panorama to start. She didn't know why she was coming to me. As the conversation developed, after twenty or thirty minutes, all body language indicated that she was more confident, and it was then that she started talking about something that worried her and limited her life: constant pain in her lower limbs. Hmm! If you have read the case of the right knee and the LED lamp, I have already given you an insight into the possible meaning of pain in the lower limbs. In this case, there was no distinction between left and right. They were both. Analysing it from a perspective of symbolism of the lower limbs, everything indicated that there was a difficulty in progressing in life. "Progression" means anything related to actions. Act. As simple as that. It would then be expected that Andreia's life would be guided more by passivity than by action and capacity for initiative.

I then suggested that she lie down on the massage table and explained that I was going to put my hands on her head and that I would be seated at the head of that massage table. I wasn't going to make any moves. My hands would be fixed. I asked her to let me know if she felt any movement or body tension. No verbal warning was necessary because, a few minutes later, the lower limbs started to shake and rotate internally (illustration 4). The toes touched, the face showed signs of suffering and, overall, Andreia seemed anxious and very restless. The upper limbs were also contracted. It was then time to join the "power of the word" and explore the origin of the pain in the lower limbs. I started by asking the limbs to relax, as I already had understood that there was "something" who wanted to communicate. From that moment on, communication would be done through dialogue.

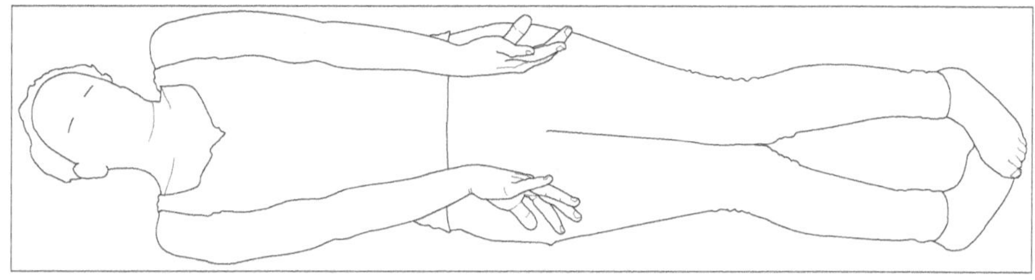

Illustration 4 – Andreia's global position was like this illustration. The most notable was the internal rotation of the thighs and the contraction of the upper limbs.

Returning to the source of the problem was a simple task. So far, everything seemed to be going well. Andreia had an "emotional cyst" since she was two years old. For some reason in today's life, these memories have come up: pain in the lower limbs and difficulty in moving. What happened then at the age of two? Andreia was in a kind of cradle and wanted to walk, but she was stuck. Her mother's voice and her words were well recorded: "Be quiet! Stop!". Well, that's what happened. Andreia was stuck with those memories and became a person without initiative power. For some life event, these memories released at 39 years of age, in the form of persistent pains. What options did I have to solve the problem? Various. I chose to take her to meet the two-year-old child (herself, with two years old) and her mother. Over the course of the session, I explored the possibility that that "weight" of the legs could disappear, through a mediation between Andreia (child and adult) and her mother. In many cases, this approach would resolve the issue. If it was a perfect resolution, like output from a troubleshooting manual. But humans are not accompanied by manuals because they are more complex. Andreia was visibly in pain, she was crying and the pain in her legs increased. It was then that she said to me: "I don't want to get rid of this weight. I want to carry it for my mother, because she can't take it!".

This option is not perfect for solving the problem. For some reason, or several, Andreia chose to stay with the pain. In order not to give too much attention to this restriction, I created conditions for the "adult Andreia" to put the "child Andreia" running and jumping. Interestingly, her mother continued to tell the child to stop, to be careful with the stairs. I asked the child to go to the stairs. Without any problem. She went up and down without difficulty. I then helped to create a form of communication between the "adult Andreia" and the "child Andreia" that would be used so that both could communicate. Weird? No. An important resource when it is necessary for the past to connect with the present, when something is not fully resolved. It seems to have been effective. Andreia's face was much more relaxed and her general body posture was open, relaxed. In my notes, I just ended with a "Fantastic". However, Andreia did not come to more sessions. I have no feedback on what happened. I can only imagine. I do not believe that Andreia had got rid of her pain, because she chose to "carry the weight" of her mother. I do not believe that this session was so effective that she would stop having pain. The doubt remains.

OTHER CASES

So far, I have addressed cases that have remained in my memory and that, in some way, have helped me to evolve. Several other cases remain to be addressed, each with its own history, story and interest. However, I reserve this subchapter to speak generically of cases that also marked me, but which, because they were so "simple", would not give a subchapter independently.

So, I start by presenting my first two cases of post-accident somatization. In the first case, a thirty-year-old man. He had constant headaches and quickly responded to my touch. Internally, in his head, he felt movements in several directions. Externally, what I felt was a kind of rapid vibration, as if it were an earthquake. The treatment for this headache was made only on the assumption that it was a headache originating from a deregulation of the cerebrospinal fluid circulation or the movement of the cranial joints. After the first session, the pain disappeared for a week. The same happened in the two sessions that followed. Then I realized that I was not getting to the source of the problem and that I would have to resort to other techniques to get more information. In the fourth session, I asked the man to lie down on the massage table. In previous sessions, treatment had been done sitting down. Once again, I sat at the head of the massage table and the bodily response went beyond my expectations. He started to shake, as was normal, but he was in more pain and his complaints increased and his eyes closed with suffering. The body movement then extended to the area of the shoulder girdle and upper limbs. It was clear that there was something specific there. Upper limbs, shoulder girdle, head. As the hypnotic trance already existed (not with words, but with my touch) I requested that those areas speak to me. So it was. The question that triggered an immediate response was: "What is your origin?". A simple, objective question, but one that does not always have a clear answer. In this case, it did. "Accident!", was the reply. That is, the source of that pain had been an accident. I continued my work, making him return to the moment before the accident. If I'm not mistaken, it was an accident that happened at the age of 22. Using the form of a television command, I clicked on the forward button, walking towards the moment of the accident. When we got to that moment, the man's body contracted violently and stayed in a constant tension, as if it was frozen. An interesting reaction. I continued to walk with the forward button, throughout the moment of the accident. The body was still tense, but it already had some movement. In that phase, I then chose to separate the present moment from the moment of the accident, making this man analyse the accident as if he were a spectator. Fortunately, it was something he managed to do well (not always happens that way), so it was also easy to continue to analyse with "different eyes" all the circumstances that led to the accident and, also, to analyse the post-accident. It was also possible for the man to be free of bodily pain, as he was, at that moment, facing traumatic moments, safely and accompanied. Since that session, he has never had a headache or scapular pain again (at least of the kind that he had in this case).

Similarly, the second case I had was of a 27-year-old woman. The accident had been more violent, so the body tension was manifested not only in the trunk, but in the lower limbs. In addition to bodily pain, there was an unspecified fear and anxiety. The treatment was guided in a very similar way to the previous case. The only exception is that, in this case, the "cure" (if we can call it that) did not occur through linguistic techniques, but it was the girl's own body that carried out the self-correcting movements. That is, there were physical restrictions that the body itself was able to correct, with non-conscious movements. Encouraged and accompanied by me, it is true, and with the surprise stamped on this woman's face, to see her body moving without her conscious will. In both cases, it was possible to make bodily pain disappear, returning to a past with physical trauma. In one case, the resolution was made with hypnosis techniques. In the other case, the resolution was made with the self-correction promoted by the woman's body.

Previously, I had already said that it was possible to "command at a distance" the body movements of the people I was treating. In the case of Sofia at about two and three meters. In the case of Nuno, about eight meters (the limit of the room where I was). These cases are *sui generis*, they are fabulous, and I constantly think that I was never prepared for such a thing to exist. At least in my training as a health professional.

There is yet another case that fascinated me and that happened with a physical therapist with whom I was taking a course. We were on a course entirely dedicated to physical treatment: osteopathy and myo-aponeurotic crocheting. In one of the intervals, the physiotherapist with whom I was training, felt his head pounding and was visibly tired. When I saw his status, I asked him if he would accept that I saw him, hoping to have another new experience and new learning. This session was fantastic. The connection time to his "non-conscious" was in less than a minute and any thought that I had of bone movement, his body reacted instantly. Something had already happened to me in a similar way, especially with the pregnancy of my first child. This case was rare due to the speed of the reactions. I just had to imagine a movement (for example, turning his head to one side) that it happened. I was surprised that the physical therapist did not ask me questions about what was happening. After all, it was not normal for this to happen! The explanation for not being surprised was the same as other sessions, with other people. Most of them think that I'm moving my hands and making the respective movements. In the case of this physiotherapist, I only had my indicator at the junction between the frontal bone and the parietal bones. Only. In the case of Sofia and Nuno, it was a few meters away. Still, they felt that it was I who performed the movements. Most people do not consider my treatment "strange", because they think that body movements are performed by me. My hands are always still (except when it is intentional to exert a corporal force). In some cases, they are not even in contact with the person being treated.

During a training I gave on my method of *body listening* – feeling the subtle movements that exist in our body – I met an acupuncture therapist. It was easier for me to teach him some concepts because he was more familiar with energy and meridian concepts. There is no need for a background in this theoretical field, but it helps to understand other concepts. What did his presence mark me in? In one of the classes, he told me: "Ricardo, I stopped doing acupuncture with needles. I just think about the point I want, and the results are identical!". The concept is like the one that got me here. At one point, I thought: "If it is possible to influence cranial movements with thought or intention, then in theory I can influence everything I want" (and that we are allowed). In the case of my trainee, his thought was: "What if I think about the acupuncture point? I will not need needles. I will just stimulate the point, mentally, as if it was a needle.". It worked. That's all that matters.

Speaking now of a more recent case. In one of my training sessions dedicated to the themes of the body and body symbolism I had a trainee – Renata – who doubted what I was saying (like what I have already discussed throughout this book). She was confused that someone could be left without voluntary control of the body. She was confused that someone could be awake (understand it as "to be conscious") and see his or her own body moving autonomously (controlled by the "non-conscious"). As usual, I prefer to demonstrate my theories. Even at the risk of the appearance of variables that still elude my comprehension. I usually invite the trainees to feel the subtle movements in each other. Let there be no illusions! The acquisition of a new type of sensitivity can be acquired quickly, but it can also be time consuming. As a rule, I use techniques that I know tend to give faster and more visible results. In this class, I kept the tradition and invited the trainees to exchange among themselves so that they could feel the subtle movements of the bodies of each one. We did some standing exercises and others on the massage table. At one point, one of the trainees called me with her eyes. It was the trainee who was with Renata! "Now here we go!", I thought, already smiling. This trainee felt movements in Renata's head and needed to know if it was that movement that was being sought. Fortunately, yes. I left her a few moments longer and gave her some guidelines by ear. The movements did not increase. They did not decrease. Renata talked to us and constantly said "I don't believe in any of this!". As we had reached an impasse, I asked the trainee at the head of the massage table to give me her place. I wanted to continue from there. By this time, all the trainees had already formed a circle around the massage table, to observe. I spent about three minutes with my hands on her head. In silence.

Renata kept the words: "I don't believe in any of this!".

At the same time, the trainees smiled and told me that she was "hard to chew". I confess that I still like to hear something similar because, from experience, I learned that the "conscious" is very different from the "non-conscious". The "hard to chew" is part of the conscious. I continued with my hands on Renata's head. I then started to see micro-expressions on her face. There were little tremors. Renata started to smile. While smiling, she continued to say: "This is not going to do anything!". When she finished her sentence, she started laughing. "It's now. There you are!", I thought. The trainees around me followed her laughter. In fact, the laughter was contagious. I wanted to laugh. Renata's body then began to give some precious indications. Her abdomen became slightly tense and there was an increase in the range of inspiration and exhalation. "Ricardo, there are restrictions in the abdomen!", was what my inner voice communicated to me. I left the head of the couch and placed my right hand in the area of the solar plexus, between the stomach and the liver, between the chest and the abdomen. The laughter increased. Renata complained about the pain it caused her but remained faithful: "I don't believe in any of this!". Once again, one of the trainees said to me: "Look, she is very rational.". To all the trainees, I remember saying to them:

"Calm. For me, Renata is like an onion. So far, I took a layer off it. Below, there will be many more.".

A minute later, Renata went from laughing to compulsive crying. The trainees stopped commenting, stopped smiling. They looked at me. The answer they got was a simple smile and an "I told you." Everything that followed from there is not something to explore. My intention was to make a demonstration and not a treatment for a specific complaint. As in all classes, in the demonstrations, there were always one or more people who discovered traumas to be resolved. In the case of Renata, and similar people, such a demonstration can have a profound impact on the way they view life. These are moments that contradict values and beliefs and that have an impact on their behaviours, but, above all, on their identity and their sense of belonging. In the film *The Rite*, a film about an allegedly true story of a Vatican exorcist, actor Anthony Hopkins tells his apprentice:

"Choosing not to believe in the devil won't protect you from him.".

If we escape the literal sense of the existence of supernatural entities, we can interpret the phrase as being said (in other ways) by different areas of knowledge: it is necessary to resolve our conflicts, it is necessary to face fears and avoid pretending that they do not exist. They will always be there, until we resolve them.

To end the chapter dedicated to presenting some standard cases that make us question the concepts of "life", "health" and "disease", I present two cases that happened with two professional athletes (I intend to leave the modalities to be identified) that I followed. The potential of the therapy that I have presented to you throughout the various cases can be applied for different purposes: seeking and resolving past traumas, communicating with certain diseases, communicating with memories lodged in the body and others. My relationship with sport is close, so much of my evolution in the field of manual therapy has taken place with the support of sporting events and professional and amateur athletes. How has touch-induced trance therapy changed my performance with athletes? Most of them have physical restrictions that limit movements, that condition plays, that condition all physical activity. Above all, they are people. They have problems like any other people. Personal problems, family problems and professional problems. In addition to the physical trauma caused by intense physical activity, we add the various traumas acquired in other ways (emotional and mental, for example). All of them condition the physical body and, directly or indirectly, will interfere with sports performance. It is appropriate to identify body restrictions that prevent full sport performance.

I remember an athlete who had a perfect self-sabotage system. He could be winning easily, but, over time, he created situations that put him at risk of losing the game. It was the way found to get energy (anger) and motivation to excel on the field and win the games. I once asked him if he had already thought about his self-sabotage cycle and why he spent so much energy creating this mechanism. I remember that, after a game, I asked him to lie down on the massage table. I had noticed that he was breathing badly. He was extremely anxious. Certainly, I thought, he would have chest restrictions. It could be from his personal life, from the opposing team or even from the referee. It could be anything. I decided to explore. I put my right hand on his chest. I just concentrated on feeling the subtle movement of the body in that area. After feeling the rhythm of the movement (restricted, in fact) I focused only on returning a broader, more flexible pattern of movement. Basically, it was to imagine that the chest expanded freely and that it moved symmetrically in all possible directions. It was a session that took about thirty minutes, but it immediately resolved an existing problem. The athlete calmed down and felt lighter and more confident. Sports therapy requires health professionals to respond quickly. I didn't solve the basic problem for him, but I did solve a temporary issue that limited him to a semi-final game that would take place in the late afternoon (it was a day with multiple competitions).

Another case was with a female athlete, also a professional. She had back pain and I, in order to start collecting information, asked her to stay upright. I put my left hand on the kidney area to feel the general body movement. Standing, it is very quick to identify body restrictions. I remember being in this position for about two minutes and feeling upward and downward movements in the kidney region. I also remember looking at the athlete's face, starting to see her go white and signalling, with my eyes, to a massage therapist who was beside me. I knew she was going to pass out. There was no time for more. The athlete fell into my arms and I only had time to support her fall. The massage therapist looked at me in surprise. The athlete was well hydrated and was not hypoglycaemic (low blood sugar). She didn't even notice she passed out. As soon as she fell on the floor, she opened her eyes, smiled and asked me: "What am I doing on the floor?". I explained that she had passed out for two seconds. I helped her to get up and she no longer had back pain. Curiously, she said to me: "Wow! It feels like I slept all night!".

This was one of the first cases that came to me and that I call them "reset".

In this case, I "reset" the kidneys. The kidney is a symbol of body energy. No wonder she felt a higher energy level. Good learning! It is possible to "reset" certain organs and energy levels.

Illustration 5 presents a simple fascial test, which is a variant of the test I performed on this athlete. However, if you do this test (at your own risk!), it is very likely that you will get a "reset".

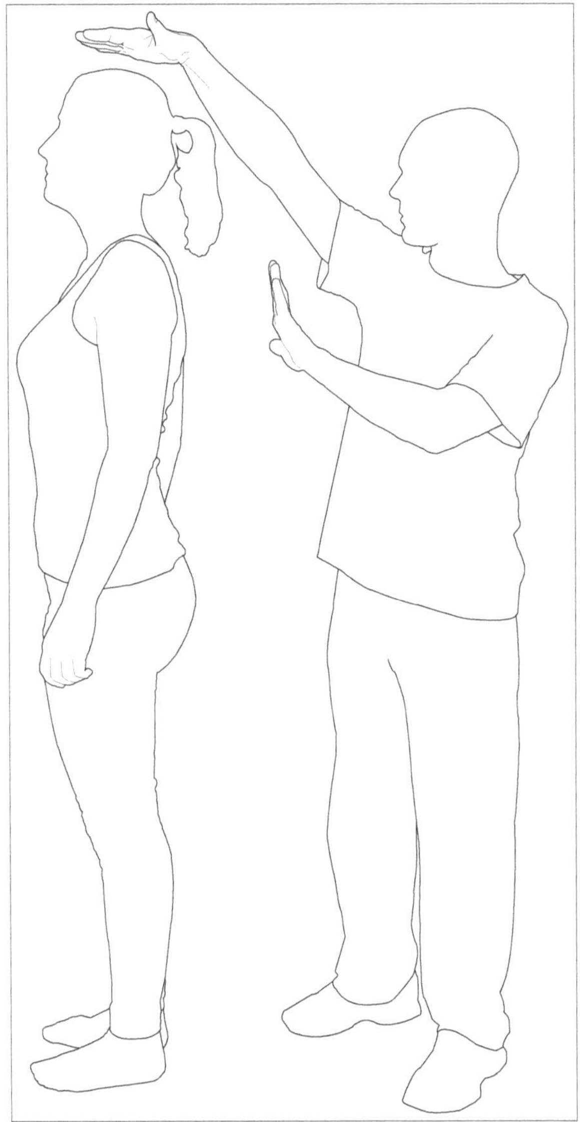

Illustration 5 – Fascial test, standing, without touching the person. This is one of my favourites and most used. If you use it, merely by copying the illustration, it is not surprising if you find manifestations like those I described in this chapter.

CHAPTER III

FROM A FREE FALL TO A PATH OF OPENNESS TO UNDERSTANDING AND ACCEPTANCE

This final chapter will serve to talk about the impact that the experiences, such as those I reported in the previous chapter, had on my life. It will also serve to talk about all areas of knowledge that influenced my perspective of therapy. Many of them scientific. Many of them are unscientific. In a first instance, I will summarize the main lessons I learned from these therapeutic experiences.

I want to make it very clear that there is no single therapy that is the answer to all problems. There is no *one model fits all* or *one size fits all*.

LEARNINGS

The lessons I learned from these therapeutic sessions are diverse, but can be summarized as follows:

1. We are made up of "parts".
2. The "parts" can be various things, from emotions, memories, repetitive cycles, cells, organs, diseases and even more than that.
3. It is possible to communicate specifically with the "parts".

4. The "parts" can manifest themselves in different ways: by body movements, by speech, by writing or even by other people who are nearby. These people act as channels of communication. I find it hard to say this, but that's what I saw.

5. The body, spirit, soul, are good by nature. Even in the most exuberant physical manifestations, such as apnea, the risk of harm to the person is zero. Physical manifestations only occur to convey a message to us.

6. The more instruments (understand it as knowledge) we master, the more opportunities we will have for successful communication with the "parts".

7. There is "something" more intelligent and capable of self-healing. As therapists, we are just "there, in that moment", assisting in a healing process. We will be more "listeners" than "prescribers". We will only be able to get results if the other person's "non-conscious" allows us to.

SEARCH FOR ANSWERS

THE CONVENTIONAL APPROACH

Nursing training gave me the basis to analyse all situations in a conventional way, from an evidence-based perspective, from a perspective of analysing scientific articles, on a "square" basis and made for the formation of the "masses". And so, it would have to be. Education of the "masses" is different from individual education. In all the experiences I reported in Chapter II, I have always tried to focus on explaining the phenomena from a scientific perspective. I say that "I tried", because it was difficult to do so, having to resort to theories called esoteric, hidden, alternatives and other similar names or concepts. The truth is that having the maximum knowledge of different areas prepares us better to obtain results (in this case, therapeutic). Conventional health training is, of course, an asset. In addition to making it easier for us to explain certain phenomena, it prepares us to be able to search for information in places with updated information, namely in scientific databases. Conventional health training prepares us for three main things (without developing concepts too much here): diagnosis, intervention and intervention evaluation. We diagnose. We intervene. We evaluate. The question of diagnosis is certainly controversial, as it is a concept that is still very much "protected" by medicine. However, whether in medicine, or in another area, "diagnosis" is the first part of an intervention: collecting information and trying to fit it in a "drawer". Basically, it's giving it a name. Apart from medicine, or non-conventional medicine, diagnosis is common to other areas, such as vocational training: the "needs analysis". Computer companies themselves make the "diagnosis" of your computer. Following the diagnosis, we have the intervention. In health, we can consider the intervention as the "treatment". Therefore, a health professional is expected to "treat" or "cure" a person. It is not to cure a "patient" or a "client". It is to heal the person. Heal from what? Well. Certainly, this will have several answers. Heal the body? The mind? Or something different? We then need to assess the intervention or interventions and monitor the evolution of the situation. The assessment may involve changing the intervention. The problem with the conventional approach lies between diagnosis and intervention/treatment. How to name something that goes beyond the traditional? I challenge you.

Find a medical book that talks about touch at a distance. In other words, a book that says that it is possible to cause body movements from "x" meters away, just with thought.

You won't find it. However, if this happens, please send me a message by e-mail and tell me that source. I will be happy to read it and "dissect it". How to name something unknown? How to "diagnose"? If this is difficult enough, then how will we act? How will we treat/cure the person? Well, I don't have an answer to give you. It is necessary to learn continuously and find the answers in several and varied sources – scientific or not. That's what I had to do. If the experiences in Chapter II made me question everything I had learned, then it was time to start looking for other paths.

OSTEOPATHY, SACRO-CRANIAL AND FASCIAL THERAPY

I have always been fascinated by manual therapy, since I took the first massage course. That is why it was natural for me to continue my training with osteopathy. To summarize osteopathy in one sentence: osteopathy is a therapy that uses the manipulation of soft tissues and the manipulation of hard tissues (bones), through *thrust* techniques, to achieve body homeostasis. In other words, it uses bone manipulations/ exercises/movements, which produce a "click" sound, to align bone structures.

However, this is a reducing view of osteopathy. This can be differentiated into three branches: structural osteopathy (the most physical part, of bone manipulation); visceral osteopathy (involving the manipulation of organs, through physical techniques) and energetic osteopathy (manipulation essentially of organs, through techniques similar to " expansion O", of which I spoke in Chapter I). Within energy osteopathy, I will include another therapy, created by John Upledger, which is sacro-cranial therapy. This therapy presupposes a tactile ability, developed in the sense of "feeling subtle movements", different from blood circulation, ventilation or the lymphatic system. It presupposes feeling the movement of the cerebrospinal fluid between the skull and the sacrum. It is, therefore, a tactile skill quite different from that developed for massage therapy or other manual therapy.

Finally, in this subchapter, I mention fascial therapy. Fascial therapy has assumptions very similar to those of sacro-cranial therapy. It presupposes feeling subtle movements, in this case the fascia. Feel the fascia and all its movements. Then let's complicate things. Almost the entire body is fascia. All body structures are interconnected by membranes, more or less thick. They all communicate with each other. Although fascial therapy is a physical therapy, it is also a therapy that can be included in energy therapy. Talking a little more about each branch of osteopathy: structural, visceral and energetic.

Structural osteopathy has fast and very good results. I quickly learned that. It was expected, because I already knew its potential. I knew that, in a very short time, I would achieve results superior to those obtained only with massage or bone manipulations, more or less conventional. The only detail for which I was not alert, was the fact that bone manipulations caused the release of repressed or "lodged" emotions in our body. Each bone seemed to have an associated emotion. I remember perfectly the first cervical manipulation (C1) I received, performed by my teacher. It must have been around 5pm. Since that time, but mostly at night, I laughed compulsively. Most of the time, in intense and (genuinely) felt laughter. Only around 10am the next day did the laughter slow down and finally stopped. "Incredible!", I thought. Since that time, I have become accustomed to seeing intense emotional releases, originating in different bones, organs and other bodily structures. Structural osteopathy helped me to understand other (physical) mechanisms and to understand that there was an associated emotional system (which was even quite specific), with emotions located in certain structures (bone or organ). Later, I realized that it was not just these structures that had associated emotions. Later, I will talk about this subject.

Visceral osteopathy. An unconventional way to treat organs. Mostly, physical techniques are used in order to improve their functioning. As with structural osteopathy, I quickly discovered that organs also have emotions associated with them. It does not occur to me to say much more about visceral osteopathy, unless we can also do it with "intention", that is, in a more energetic perspective.

Things change when we talk about sacro-cranial therapy and fascial therapy. It changes because, in addition to being something more specific, it is something that brings together structural osteopathy and visceral osteopathy. To imagine that we have a subtle movement, which differs both from the circulatory system, as well as from the respiratory or lymphatic system and has its own rhythm, is something for which I had no basis to understand. "How can we feel such a movement?", I often asked myself. Well. With the development of a sensitivity for which I had no training yet. Simply "feel", or as they say in fascial therapy: *listening*. This *listening* is not listening related to hearing. It is not auditory. It is to appeal to synaesthesia (in the global sense of the senses), to "listen" to the body. I draw attention to the fact that synaesthesia differs from kinaesthesia (which refers only to touch). Sacro-cranial therapy presupposes feeling the movement of cerebrospinal fluid, which waves at its own pace between the skull and sacrum, through the neural tube, following the central nervous system. Sceptical, as I usually am, I searched scientific sources to find out if there were studies in this field. There were and there are, but they are scarce and inconsistent. However, they shared common conclusions. With the same "guinea pigs", different therapists identified different "sacro-cranial" rhythms.

This fact did not surprise me, nor does it surprise me. Making a parallel with massage therapy, I always found articles that stated that massage did not have any effects, be it an increase in body temperature, an increase in venous return, or an increase in endorphins, among others. What I knew was not true. Massage has many good effects. Of course, as in other professional areas, it will depend on the professional who performs it and on their own personal characteristics and the level of technical instruction (theoretical and practical).

If the sacro-cranial rhythm is not "a certain thing" or "evident", then what movements should we feel? As I learned throughout the course, the movement of the cerebrospinal fluid was related to the movements of the cranial and sacrum bones. If you want to study the amount of bones in the skull, I wish you luck. They are immense: frontal, parietal, occipital, temporal, sphenoid, ethmoid, vomer, mandible, nasal, lacrimal, nasal conchae, zygomatic, palatal. Ufff! Each of them with its own "flexion" and "extension" movement (opening and closing), based on the rhythm of the cerebrospinal fluid. To give just one example, fast rhythms can indicate hyperactivity and slow rhythms can indicate depression. Flexion and extension must have similar amplitudes and, if they do not, we must promote this similarity, with specific techniques.

There are interesting points in sacro-cranial therapy, but what most attracted me (and attracts me) is that the techniques used were not exactly physical, but energetic. Simply, with a very soft and superficial touch, we should perform the body *listening*, in specific areas, feeling the movement of the structures. That is why not only the bones were felt, but also the entire fascia. The correction (the therapeutic effect) did not occur mechanically/physically. No. We just had to be with our hands still and, with our mind (with our thought!!!), imagine that we were correcting the movements of the bones or fascia. To imagine! With our "intention". In illustration 6, for example, we have the placement of hands on the hyoid and on the frontal bone, already on the border with the nasal bone.

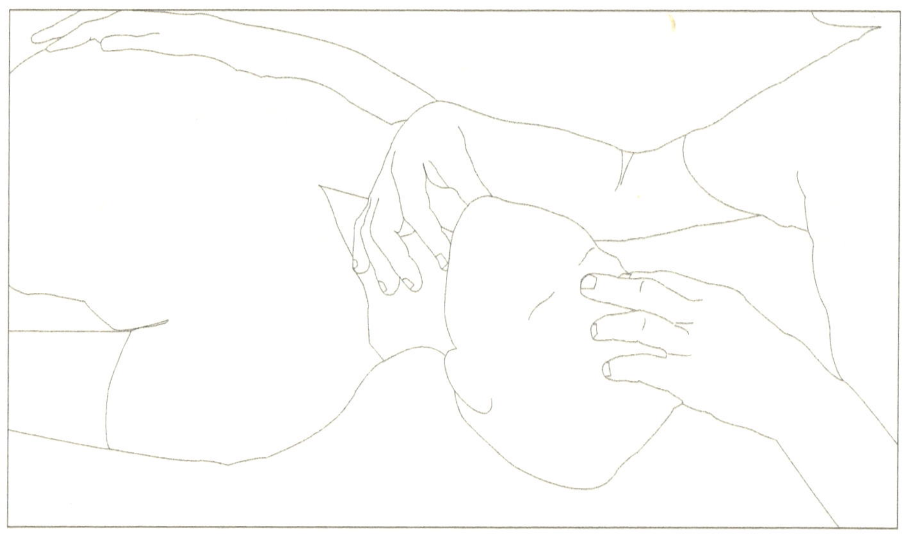

Illustration 6 – This position, which is based on a real treatment, allowed movements in all cranial bones. Through "intention".

Before proceeding with what I consider to be the main idea – the "intention" – I would like to mention that, throughout the course, I had received some treatments carried out by my teacher. The truth is that I saw his hands still, but I literally felt my body moving internally. On the right flank of the abdomen, the sensation was very similar to the detachment of leaves, one by one. I also felt my head "inflating" and "deflating". What a strange feeling! It was like someone was touching my brain directly. That fascinated me! It still fascinates, but no longer with the typical enthusiasm of the first time.

Returning to "intention". If, with the mind, and with our thoughts, we could influence the movement of the bones... then...!

"Ricardo! If this is possible (and it even seems to work), then you will be able to communicate with every part of the body!".

Well, the truth is: yes, it is possible to communicate with all the "parts" that we want. Whether they are more or less evident, whether we are aware of them or not. In his books, John Upledger mentions the existence of an "internal doctor", a "greater conscience" who will know how to heal itself. Our intention should be to "talk" with this "internal doctor", in order to obtain results. Initially, I used this concept in therapeutic practice. I still use it occasionally. I use it whenever I am in doubt which "part" I will address. Not all are specific. Not all have the same name. Not all want to make themselves known. I learned that the "parts" are not only physical, but also emotional (or "emotional cysts", as Upledger calls it), memories of current life, memories of other generations, among many others. I even came across a person who had more than two "entities" talking at the same time. I had never seen that before. It is true that I remembered the films of exorcism and demonic possession, but I never let myself be carried away by these thoughts. I chose to consider that there were several "memories" to communicate at the same time. They interrupted each other. They talked to each other, quickly, emotionally and forcefully. What a mess! It looked like I was surrounded by people talking at the same time. But not. There was only one person in front of me.

I started to develop a new way of working. From there, I would have to be incisive. Determined. Imposing rules. I started talking to the "parts", independently, acting as a pivot between them all. Basically, a conflict mediator. Sometimes there was only a "part" talking, sometimes another. Sometimes they spoke only to me, sometimes they spoke to each other.

There was a situation that scared me, and I talked about it before. It was in the situation where one of the "parts" chose to use someone else to communicate with me. No. I didn't like that moment. I dealt with it with determination and enforced rules. I believe that that person was the best "vehicle" to communicate with me, at that moment. It's all right. I even accept that. What I do not accept is that it is without the consent (conscience) of the person to whom this happens. This paragraph already has (very) controversial information and indicates other subjects that are taboo. That's enough for now.

I have not always resolved the conflicts arising from these interactions with the "non-conscious" or the "parts", in a very directive and firm way. I learned how to do it. The results improved and I started to communicate better and without so many physical manifestations. I started to understand what was "told".

The sacro-cranial therapy changed the way I see, hear, feel and understand the world. Just because I dared to use some of its concepts to go further.

COACHING, NEUROLINGUISTIC PROGRAMMING AND HYPNOSIS

Throughout the sessions I attended, the physical manifestation of somato-emotional releases was always visible. I saw everything. People turning pale, grey, almost as if they were dead; to stop ventilating (breathing); to exuberant dilation of veins, as if they were going to explode; to body twists that I never thought possible. Everything triggered by touch and *listening* (the time to wait for "non-conscious" communication). However, underlying all these manifestations, there was always a great doubt and a great concern. I didn't understand many of the physical manifestations and I needed to understand them. These only provided me with some data. For example, I could detect the "eventual" location of a problem, if the abdomen moved. I could interpret it symbolically, but it was very reductive. I needed to communicate in the most obvious way I knew: using the word. I needed to speak directly with the "parts", and I needed to hear the answer. Or read, as happened in the case of the "writing shoulder". For this, I felt the need to develop other skills: knowing how to communicate better. To have more communication tools. In this sense, I chose to carry out training cycles in several areas. Two of these areas, which, meanwhile, became fashionable, were coaching and neurolinguistic programming.

The training was extremely expensive. In fact, much more expensive than a doctorate or a master's degree. In terms of academic recognition, it was/ is zero. Even so, I do not regret having done it, even after having done it in Lisbon, with all the extra living and travel expenses (I am from Porto). I took three courses: Business coaching, NLP Practitioner and NLP Master.

Now, what is coaching and neurolinguistic programming? Basically, it is "everything" and "nothing". They are techniques used in different media and for different purposes. They can either be used to improve the techniques of psychology and psychoanalysis, or they can be used for marketing and advertising, for the creation of political speeches or even for "brainwashing". Therefore, anyone will use the techniques based on their professional/personal background, according to their interests. There are hundreds (if not thousands) of techniques. Fortunately, the courses had a great deal of practicality, which made me evolve a lot.

The practice was almost always done using people outside the course. They were dozens. From that practice, and since then, I have identified techniques for which I see no use and others in which I see a lot of potential. In practical terms, however, they all bring results. It will always depend on who we have ahead of us. In addition to the courses, I invested a lot in books and in knowing different approaches, in the therapeutic sense. Overall, neurolinguistic programming has changed the way I analyse and interact with the world. For my father, he would say it was harmful to me. I feel like I benefited. It is true that I recognize what my father tries to convey to me. On the one hand, it took away my spontaneity (which is very necessary!) and made me more analytical (it has reinforced a personal characteristic). After all, with the tools that that training gave me, I started to identify more quickly who lied to me, who manipulated me, who really had an interest in talking or being with me, who ignored me or who enjoyed me. Intuitively, I already knew it. With more objective tools, things flowed faster. It had its negative side, it is true. It also had its positive side, namely in the management of my own company, in the management of multiple networks of contacts and in interpersonal relationships.

The neurolinguistic programming helped me a lot to understand how to communicate better with the "parts" that manifested themselves during the sessions described in Chapter II. With the techniques learned, I was able to communicate with the word, with the conversation, as I did daily with anyone. With neurolinguistic programming, I understood something that, only later, I would come to realize I started to understand the way of building a hypnotic process, namely the processes based on Milton Erickson. There are different hypnotic approaches. The "Ericksonian hypnosis" is not always the most accepted or considered "the best", but it still brought results. I was unable to develop more methods of hypnosis because most of the training was in London and I did not have the time and financial resources to do it. Still, I wish I had. The more tools we have, the better.

When I started to dedicate myself to studying and practicing hypnosis (of course, I am not going to say that I am a hypnotherapist!), I also consulted some hypnotherapists. To learn their methods and to solve personal cases. I was disappointed, overall. Some used scripts. I was lying on the couch or on a *chaise longue*, listening to the sheets of paper turning, as the therapist read me what was written there. In an automatic and monotone speech, as if each person were the same. Others used techniques without scripts but used a scheme so "predictable" that it felt like they were taking me where they wanted to go and not where I should be going. It was difficult to abstract myself. All the training that I had and that continued to develop, allowed me to understand all that script. In the neighbourhood, much of the hypnotic approach was done with Milton Erickson's principles and the neurolinguistic programming gave me the basis to understand and adapt it to each person.

As for hypnosis, I did some punctual training, taught by Americans. Once again, I understood the entire script. I saw many people following it "to the letter", but I dissected them to identify the key points of the strategy used. It was not very difficult. Overall, it comes down to:

1. Induce trance (by touch or by words).
2. Guide the person to a safe place to start a "trip" (to the past, for example) and also to bring that person to this place, in case "something" gets out of hand.

3. Taking the person to the past (or the future!), to a trauma, to a past life (wow! What did I say!) or others.
4. Solve the problem at the source: in childhood? In intrauterine life? In a previous life? Or is it something from the future that has not yet happened? (ouch! There I am abusing again!).
5. Bring the person to the safe place.
6. Bring the person to the present, to the "here and now".

I don't always follow this scheme. Sometimes I am more direct. I take the person more quickly to a trauma and then I manage what appears to me. Sometimes, I create the "safe haven". It depends on my intentions and the people I follow. Trance induction has been something I've always been able to do with touch, since Susana (see Chapter II). With hypnosis or with neurolinguistic programming techniques, I learned to communicate with all those "parts" that wanted to communicate with me. The physical manifestations began to decrease, comparing to some years ago. When they come, I immediately try to talk to them. Basically, what I say to the "parts" is that I do not understand only the physical manifestations, so I request authorization to communicate with them through the word or through writing. That "part" will now use the mouth, or the hand, of the person being "treated". It is funny then to see the person talking or gesturing or writing, without being able to have voluntary control. Attention! People are conscious! They can see and hear themselves, but they can't control their body. Consciousness is only to contemplate what is said by the "non-conscience". It is strange, but it is a fantastic world! There are cases in which there is no authorization to communicate by speech. No problem! It is done through writing, drawing or gestures. There is almost always a way to communicate. Except when the "non-conscious" forbids any attempt of contact. That often happens. Simply, at that time and place, I am not the right person to solve a problem. However, I can ask for suggestions on who can solve it: massage therapist, doctor, nurse, psychologist, nutritionist or other? Just enumerate.

Neurolinguistic programming and hypnosis. Without knowing it, in the case of Sofia (see Chapter II), I used a perfect hypnosis protocol. At the time, it came naturally to me. Without knowing the theory on the subject. Without techniques. It was the most perfect I've done so far.

BODY LANGUAGE

Inevitably, in order to understand the reasons for certain emotions to be located more in a tissue or an organ, or in another "part", it is important to understand body language. Body language is not a "science". I would say that it will be rather an "art", which is closely related to symbolism. There are several books on body language. Some more complete than others. Some even seem completely wrong. Others are inspiring. In any case, there are always areas of convergence between all. Obviously, I am not going to talk exhaustively about body language, but just to mention that body language is extremely important to obtain results like those described in Chapter II. It is also extremely useful to combine the study of body language with the concept of *chakras*. I will show the relationship between the two. It is also useful to watch the *Lie to Me* television series. For a practical sense, I will address body language by dividing the body into:

1. Two halves, in the sagittal plane (right and left).
2. Four parts: lower limbs, upper limbs, trunk and head.

Starting with the body halves – right and left. Symbolically, our right side of the body is related to the father/male figure and the future. That is, it is related to a father, a brother, a grandfather, an uncle, a friend, a boyfriend, or another man. It is also related to the future and "where we are going" and "where we want to go". Our left side is related to the maternal/female figure and the past. It relates to a mother, a sister, a grandmother, an aunt, a friend, a girlfriend, or another woman. It relates to the past and "where we came from". All of this, in an extremely simplistic way. There are books that refer to this symbolism in the opposite way. They do it wrong, by my experience.

What is the practical interest of the right side or the left side of the body, from a therapeutic point of view? Easy! Think about this detail: in your professional practice (I presume that in the health area) or in your personal life (family or friends), how many people did you find that only get injured on the left or right side of the body? For example, they only get injured on the left foot, the left knee, the left elbow, or the left hemiface? Or vice versa. Only injuries on the right side. Never happened to you? Never noticed? Or did you notice and never gave great importance to the case? Do you think it was a coincidence? No, it was not.

There is a relationship between the right/left sides and injuries or illness. It is a symbolic relationship. It is a form of "collective non-conscious" communication, using the body, using the material, the physical.

To interpret these signals, we must understand what each region of the body represents. For example, pain in the left knee may indicate a relationship that has been poorly managed in the past, a conflict with a mother figure, an inflexibility of thought or a resistance to accepting to change something in life. A mother who won't let us evolve? A girlfriend and a relationship that has already "ended", and that it is necessary to move on? Actions that we know we must take in the present moment, but that we don't like, and that we insist on not accepting to change them? Rigidity of thought and inflexibility with past issues that relate to a female figure? Another example: right shoulder. Weight of responsibility. Is there anything in life that is taking me to carry the "weight", the "burden" of my father, brother, uncle or friend? If so, then it is time to change something, as the body started somatising. Through pain, or loss of functionality, it became evident that there is a problem that needs to be solved.

In addition to the right/left side, it is necessary to understand what each body zone represents: lower limbs, upper limbs, trunk and head. The lower limbs represent body movement, locomotion, escape, "walking forward". They represent our ability to move from x to y, from one place to another. Symbolically, the legs represent our ability to act, to move forward in life, to act according to our desires and motivations and the ability to survive. Faced with a threat, do we flee or counterattack? Any problem that arises in the lower limbs, namely pain or lack of strength, represents an inconsistency between what "we think we should do" and what "we are really doing".

In the lower limbs, we can be more specific and identify the feet, knees and hips as key points for interpreting the origin of "emotional cysts". The feet represent locomotion. The ability to walk. Injuries, pain or lack of strength in the feet mean that the person is encountering too many obstacles in life and is trying to overcome them in a wrong or hasty way. Basically, it indicates that the person must readjust the time of the proposal to solve a problem or move on to a project. It means the person must slow down. If someone tells me: "Ah, but player *x* has pain in his left foot, because he had a trauma due to the "slide tackle" of another player!". I reply: "Okay. Right. It is a physical trauma. But nothing guarantees that this trauma does not have a symbolic relationship.". You will notice that there are athletes who only suffer injuries on one side of the body (either right or left). And it is not a coincidence, nor does it have anything to do with muscle chains maladjustments. When you see this, remember: you may be facing a form of non-verbal, symbolic communication that may require other forms of treatment than just physical treatment. For the better or for the worst, physical treatment is done. However, it may have short-term effects. I strongly believe that you will recognize this pattern in the people you follow (if you are a therapist) or in a family member or friend.

Now speaking of the knees. The knees are an interesting joint. Very interesting. The somato-emotional releases from these structures are usually very exuberant. Sometimes "aggressive". The knees are places full of symbolism. For example, kneeling at Mass is a sign of the importance of this joint. Kneeling is giving in. It is accepting. It is surrendering. It is to trust. It is being flexible. It is "letting it flow". Therefore, any knee problem is a sign of stiffness and inflexibility. It is a sign of obstinacy and stubbornness. It is wanting to maintain a rhythm of life, or life choices, contrary to what we need and aspire. It is refusing to change the trajectory of our life, refusing to make changes. It is to delay the actions that we know are necessary. If there is pain or lack of strength in the left knee, it is a sign that we do not want to move forward in life and that we are afraid of the future. So, we prefer to stay in the past. It can also be a rigid attitude related to a female figure. If the pain or lack of strength is in the right knee, it may represent the insecurity of the future, feeling that we are ill-prepared to face challenges or that we do not have the skills to overcome obstacles in life. It can also be a problem inherent to a male figure (father, brother, grandfather, uncle, or another man).

Moving on to the hip. Ouch! The hip. Like the knee, the hip is a complex structure and can have many problems. Such is its complexity – muscles, tendons, ligaments, vessels, nerves, bones – that it is better to analyse the hip in its entirety. The hip establishes a crucial link between the trunk (with all its vital organs) and the lower limbs. Establishes the relationship between "Heaven" and "Earth". It establishes the connection between our motivations/desires/thoughts and our action. Any problem that arises in the hip represents the difficulty in moving forward in life, it represents a repression of emotions, the postponement of projects, the inability or voluntary (but unwanted) postponement of putting into practice what is considered necessary. Here are located all the emotions of people who feel they are "losing ground", who feel insecure, who feel they are not able to move forward in life and overcome obstacles. It is like feeling "trapped" in themselves (especially in terms of the will to act and not doing it). The existence of problems in the hip can indicate the existence of serious internal challenges and conflicts, especially between the "ideal" and the "real" (the path that the person is really taking). The treatment involves aligning values, or beliefs, with the actions the person takes. It is a work of alignment between the environment, behaviour, skills, values/beliefs, identity and the sense of belonging. Whoever has training in coaching and neurolinguistic programming will quickly understand these concepts. Working on the hip emotions is a challenge that can lead to long follow-up sessions.

Speaking of the upper limbs. The upper limbs are the performers of various tasks, other than locomotion. They allow us to perform fine movements, detailed tasks and they play an important role in the defence of vital organs. Let's see, if you are distracted while I throw you a ball, what will be your instinctive reaction? You will use your upper limbs to prevent the ball from hitting you in the torso, or in the head. Simple, isn't it? In martial arts, the upper limbs are the body zones of choice for defence and attack. The function is to protect vital organs. Hence, body language is essential to understanding the person. Arms crossed in front of the torso, together with shoulders gathered over the chest (cupped protection) indicate a person who is highly protective of his or her "self", of his or her emotions and feelings. It is someone who protects himself/herself from the outside (aggressions, for example). As with the lower limbs, we can divide the upper limbs into three parts: hands, elbows and shoulders. Strangely, from my experience, except for the shoulders, I don't have much to write about hands and elbows. The hands are related to the details and the accomplishment of tasks. Like the knees, the elbows relate to the flexibility and rigidity with which we perform everyday tasks. Now, if we talk about the shoulder, it does have a different importance (in the sense of somato-emotional releases) than the hand or the elbow.

The shoulder is the pivot of the entire upper limb. It is what "bears the burden", what bears the "weight", mainly of responsibility. Pain in the shoulders and shoulder girdle indicates that we carry the burden of our own or others' responsibility. Perhaps because we are involved in more activities than we can do. Perhaps because we are perfectionists and want to be good at everything. Perhaps because we have someone in charge (children and parents, for example). As an example, it is common to see a child somatising the stroke of a parent. That is, to behave as if he/she too had had a stroke and had a hemiplegia. Simply because the person "replaces" the other and starts to carry the "burden" for him/her. Communicating with the "non-conscious" of the shoulder can be easier through writing than through speaking. The shoulder is closely related to the head and the upper chest, so it is prudent to carefully assess any communication with this structure. What does the shoulder really want to convey to us? In general, emotions are related to tasks not completed and actions that have not been initiated, but that need to be done. Procrastination leads to a lot of pain in this region.

Trunk. A complex body zone, containing numerous structures. Each of them, with an associated emotion. Dividing the trunk into two parts: the abdomen and the chest. The abdomen contains organs such as the ovaries, uterus, prostate, small intestine and large intestine, bladder, pancreas, stomach, kidneys and, to some extent, the spleen.

The ovaries and the uterus are related to reproduction and any problems in these structures may be due to fear of not leaving offspring, fear of establishing relationships with a partner, emotional self-sabotage (for example, a woman who was a victim of sexual abuse may not want to become pregnant for several traumatic reasons, with her self-image being affected). The prostate is related to the male reproductive system. Like the ovaries and the uterus, any problems in the reproductive organs may indicate the fear of abandonment, the fear of being "judged", the search for affection, safety and protection. Strangely, from my experience, I don't remember having "spoken" to the prostate. That is why I cannot develop much more than this.

As for the intestine. The small intestine and the large intestine are related to the way we face reality and "digest" the day-to-day events. It relates directly to the stomach. The intestine acts as a huge "retainer" of emotions, which means that various emotions can "lodge" in these organs. In general, any problem in the intestine leads us to people with a high need for protection and security, obstinate people, sometimes obsessive, rigid, sometimes theatrical, exaggerated and with a great need to speak. From my experience, it is almost a Russian roulette to address the emotions of these structures. We never know what is there. However, whatever the therapeutic approach, somato-emotional releases often result in "cleansing of the intestine", either with increased frequency of dejections (body waste) or with diarrhoea. It is a manifestation of physical liberation, but also emotional. The gut is indirectly related to fear: fear of the future, fear of not being perfect, fear of obstacles in life, fear of losing money, among others. It is a generic fear, related to the management of day-to-day events.

As I said, the intestine is related to the stomach. This is one of the main organs that performs digestion. From a symbolic point of view, it is the organ that makes the digestion of the day-to-day life, of all our experiences, of all the interactions we have with the outside environment and with relationships with other people. The stomach manifests itself in moments of enormous stress, especially in cases of ending of relationships. In these cases, the person cannot accept the end of that same relationship, so he/she begins to somatise through nausea, vomiting or abdominal pain. He or she may even start to reject food, going through a great weight loss period. Frustration in life? Stomach.

Now analysing the kidneys. The kidneys are related to body energy and even to existence itself. Water is their fuel. Do you drink a lot of water? It's because your energy is too much, but it runs out quickly. You may have to dose that energy better or get more supplies. Extremely dynamic people, whether physically or mentally, need to be constantly drinking water. The kidneys have an associated emotion: fear. It is not a generic fear, as in the case of the intestine. It is a concrete fear. It is the fear of dying. It is the fear of not leaving offspring. It is existential fear. The kidneys are fantastic organs, in which it is possible to perform the "reset", as in the case described in Chapter II, in "Other cases". It is our "switch". Do you want to perform a "reset" or "shut-down" like it happened to this athlete? Approach the kidneys as the first choice. You may not have permission from the "internal doctor" to do so. It doesn't hurt to ask! Do not be alarmed if the person remains "off" for a while without answering. It's normal.

In a similar way to the prostate, strangely, when writing this paragraph, I realize that I do not find memories of people who have had somatizations in the bladder, pancreas or spleen. It is weird. Either way, I generally approach the symbolism of each area. The bladder is related to control, guilt, obedience, submission and shyness. These relationships have been developed since childhood. From an early age, we are educated to control urine and any signs of incontinence, although natural in childhood, are seen socially as a reprehensible act that must be avoided. However, as I have little experience with somato-emotional releases from this organ, I can add little more. As for the pancreas and spleen, my experience is also limited. Still, there are strong relationships between these organs and the stomach, liver and intestine. Therefore, like the gut, they are organs that are not specific in terms of emotions. However, they seem to be affected by high levels of tension (read "stress", in the popular sense of the term) and by situations that are usually attributed to the stomach, such as the "digestion" of everyday situations, frustration with life, non-acceptance of ending of relationships, non-acceptance of the death of a family member or friend, confrontation with domestic violence, pessimism, deep sadness or any other trauma. If we relate to the liver, we add the emotion of anger.

The thorax houses vital structures. They are quite a few, but I will only mention those structures that "harbour" specific emotions, such as the liver, lungs and heart. These three organs are important in terms of emotions and their manifestation. They are a priority in the search for "parts" who want to communicate. We then have three important organs, which function as authentic "sponges" when it comes to absorbing emotions.

The liver is an organ associated with anger. The liver manifests itself in all those situations that "irritate" us, and in those that "we explode". From my experience, the liver is an excellent organ for looking for "emotional cysts". It is an excellent organ for somato-emotional releases, which usually result in somewhat frightening manifestations. The energy contained in these "cysts" or "parts" is associated with anger. Don't be surprised if someone jumps at you or insults you or tries to attack you. Remember: it is normal in this organ. It has nothing to do with you. They are just energetic releases, related to trauma or life experiences.

Now passing to the lungs. I have yet to find the right word to describe the main emotion of the lung. In English, it is grief. In Portuguese, it is not easy to summarize it in one word. This grief is related to grief, pain, nostalgia, longing and a sense of loss. Like the liver or heart, the lungs retain many experiences and traumas. Most of the time, the manifestations are even evident to the "naked eye". A person who is constantly coughing? Who is constantly sighing? Someone who feels like a "tightness in my chest, that even takes my breath away"? Yes, it's the lungs.

Now speaking of the heart. The heart is an organ related to life and passion. It is normal to see advertisements, associating "life" to the heart. It is also normal to associate it with Valentine's Day. Usually, we associate this heart with the colour red. Have you ever painted a heart of another colour? Wasn't it weird? The heart is an emotional "sponge" and is associated with a sense of belonging and with loving and being loved. All life experiences that affect "love" and "belonging" will cause damage to the heart. What damage?

Well, that's easy. How many people do you know who complain about "my chest hurts" or "I feel a tightness in my chest" when they end a relationship? When they are abandoned? When they lose their parents? How many people enter the hospital with chest pain and leave the hospital only with a diagnosis of "anxiety"? This heartache is very real. It means that the heart has absorbed more energy (traumatic emotions, in this case) than it can dissipate. Result? From simple chest pain to death. Yes. The heart can stop, if that accumulated energy is too high. Believe that it will not have any relation with another type of existing pathology. Simply, in a "completely healthy" person (if that exists at all), the heart may stop for lack of love and/or for lack of a sense of belonging. As for the heart, I recently read a journalistic article that described exactly what I am transmitting here. In this specific case, the news portrays Mexican children trying to enter the United States of America. Read and analyse what is described. When I read the news, I was sad, because I see the clear manifestations of what "emotional cysts" are and their somatization and I see the inability of professionals to get to the source of the problem. It is necessary to "speak" directly to the heart (if you happen to open the book on this page, please read everything I wrote back, to understand the context). It is necessary to appeal to the "internal doctor". It takes a lot. Which unfortunately, in 2019, I still don't see.

In *RTP Notícias*, September 5, 2019

"I can't feel my heart". It is the chilling appeal of some of the children who were separated from their parents during the Trump administration's strict immigration policy last year, called "Zero Tolerance".

At the border between Mexico and the USA, federal authorities separate children from their parents, family members or other adults accompanying them on the crossing. Adults are sent to federal prisons, and children and babies, in turn, are placed under the supervision of the Department of Health and Human Services.

*This separation is far from harmless, considers a report by the Department of Health and Human Services, released this Wednesday. Children, many of them victims of trauma situations in their countries of origin or resulting from the painful trip to the USA, showed **more fear, feelings of abandonment and symptoms of post-traumatic stress (PSS) than children who were not separated from their families**.*

*In addition to these psychological consequences, some children even suffer from physical symptoms due to mental trauma. "We heard a lot of **'my chest hurts'**, despite everything being fine physically," revealed one of the doctors interviewed by the researchers. Children describe psychological symptoms as "every heartbeat hurt," or "I can't feel my heart".*

These symptoms do not only appear in childhood, they often extend into adulthood. As children, they suffer from night terrors, separation anxiety and concentration problems. As adults, they face greater risks of mental and physical challenges, from depression to cancer.

*The process of reunification, considered chaotic, only added cause for concern. Some children cried, heartbroken. Some were furious and confused. **"Other children revealed feelings of fear and guilt and were concerned about their parent's well-being"**, says the report.*

***"We will have this weight on our conscience for the rest of our lives"**. The Department of Health and Human Services report is the first in-depth study on the consequences for children's mental health of the policy of separation from families, advocated by the Trump Administration. It was based on interviews with* *about a hundred mental health doctors who maintained regular interactions with children. The report covers a period of last year when the facilities were overcrowded.".*

Head. When I speak of the head, I mean the neck, face and skull and all the inherent structures, such as the brain. In terms of body language, we know that the face is rich in micro-expressions. It will then seem logical to state that it is on the face that we will find a lot of non-verbal information. Wrong! The face is rich in micro-expressions, but it is also the one we most quickly hide from the world. How? Makeup, for example. Conscious manipulation of many of our expressions. Suppression of physical manifestations. The face is easily trained to cheat. Just watch the TV presenters. They falsify expressions. However, the head covers much more than the face. As it is not my goal to be talking about body language in detail (there are so many books about it), I will talk about just a few details. All organs have specific functions that converge with the associated emotions. For example, the stomach performs digestion, and, on an emotional level, it is what "digests" everyday events and manages frustration or non-acceptance of certain events. In the head, this connection is similar.

Let us look at the neck, the mouth, the nose and the ears. The neck and mouth are closely related. They are related to oral expression. They represent what we want to "say" to the world. In order to function well and there are no "problems" in these areas, we will have to be consistent with our "essence" and the way we communicate. That would be so, in an ideal world. That doesn't exist. Daily, as we move from childhood to adulthood, we repress our expressions. We do this by "swallowing" what we don't like to hear, for example. This swallowing is related to the mouth, neck and stomach. We retain things we don't want to say: either because they are going to hurt someone, or because they are going to harm us, or for some other reason. We then start to communicate in other ways, not always aligned with our will. Then the physical manifestations of diseases begin to appear: problems with the thyroid, problems with the nose (rhinitis, for example), problems with swallowing food ("food is hard to swallow"), difficulty in oral communication, among many others. Body language helps us a lot to decipher messages from these areas. The hand in front of the mouth? Someone who is avoiding talking. In the neck? Someone who does not like what he/she is listening to and wants to express an opposite opinion but cannot for fear of reprisals. A person constantly coughing? Choking? All of these are indicators that something is not going well in the person's expression.

In the nose, the manifestations are more related to doubt, uncertainty and non-acceptance. For example, in Portuguese we have expressions like "chegar a mostarda ao nariz" ("getting the mustard to the nose") or "não me cheira bem" ("doesn't smell right"), that represent the symbolism of this area. Ears. "I don't want to hear," or "I didn't like what I heard" symbolize this area of the body. The same goes for the eyes. Gestures that protect the eyes or frown reveal that the person "does not want to see" or "is not seeing". I will not go into more detail about the head, as it is easier to do so when I speak now of the *chakras* and body symbolism.

I have no training in acupuncture, but I recognize that it is ideal for understanding how body energy works between different organs. A more simplistic way of perceiving it is through the *chakras*. These are energy centres that are in specific areas of the body and that are represented by specific symbols and colours. Classically, seven *chakras* are identified, but there are books that identify more than two dozen of them. Anyway, there are theories for all tastes. I am a fan of the *seven-chakra* theory: root, sacral, solar plexus, heart, throat, third eye and crown. If we understand only the basic concept of each *chakra*, or energy centre, together with interpretations of body language, we will quickly be able to gauge a person's "state of mind". In any of the *chakras*, it is easy to visualize the "problems". The person will tend to hide or protect them, either with their hands or with clothes or with accessories (such as backpack, suitcases, or other objects).

The *root chakra* is an energy centre located in the coccyx area and is associated with the colour red. It is located at the lower end of the spine. For this reason, it is considered the base *chakra*, linked to survival, material security and independence. If the person has problems in this area, he/she will quickly "cover" the area of the genitals with his/her hands, with an object, with more clothes (for example, a longer nightgown that reaches up to the thighs) or even with an internal rotation of the thighs.

The *sacral chakra* is located a little higher, at the level of the navel. It is associated with the colour orange and represents pleasure and sexuality. It is also related to self-esteem. This *chakra* is a "reservoir of energy". This is where the energy flows from. Just analyse yoga or martial arts or meditation and notice the common point. The control is done by breathing (in this specific case, it is more ventilatory mechanics). Even at the conventional level, respiratory rehabilitation takes place at the abdominal level, with training of the diaphragm. Any sign of blockage of this *chakra* – covering the abdomen with hands or objects or clothing – will indicate problems in terms of sexuality and the relationship with others, in a more intimate perspective. It may also indicate a lack of energy. People with problems in this *chakra* may have a white or black body colour. This shade comes from the kidneys: lack of energy or "bad energy".

The *solar plexus chakra* is located between the abdomen and the chest, in the area of the xiphoid appendix, and is associated with yellow colour. At this level, organs such as the liver and stomach are located, so this *chakra* is associated with the emotions of these organs. Basically, it is the way we "digest" the world. It is the interaction between "us and the world". Any indicator of blockage of this *chakra* leads us to a person who may be frustrated, unable to accept life events, a person who is sad, angry, hated or disappointed. The yellow of the *chakra* is visible in the person's overall tone. The person looks yellow. It is not jaundiced! It is simply a colour that tends to be more yellow. This yellow is more associated with the stomach and pancreas. The green colour is associated with the liver and gallbladder. Usually, people who have this body tone (tendency green) are associated with the Portuguese expression "tem maus fígados" ("to have bad livers"), that is, bad temper.

The *heart chakra* is in the chest and is associated with one of these colours: green or pink. This energy centre is important because it functions as a pivot between the upper *chakras* (throat, third eye and crown) and the lower chakras (root, sacral and solar plexus). The upper *chakras* are considered as "Heaven" and the lower *chakras* as "Earth". In general, "Heaven" represents the connection to the divine, our connection to a global consciousness and our intuition. The "Earth" represents the way we materialize our ideals, our thoughts and our intuition. The *heart chakra* makes the connection between "Heaven" and "Earth", so any inconsistency between our ideal and the way we materialize it will disturb this energetic centre. It is extremely vulnerable to inconsistencies between our desires, impulses or intuition and the way we express ourselves with the outside world. Shortness of breath or chest tightness are common symptoms of deregulation of this energy centre. A person with a more "reddish" skin tone is a person who has a very active energy centre. He/she is a sensitive and passionate person, but also a person who needs to be "fuelled" constantly with affection.

The *throat chakra* is an energy centre located in the neck and is associated with a blue or turquoise colour. This energetic centre separates the spiritual world from the physical world. To some extent, it works similarly to the *heart chakra*, separating "Heaven" and "Earth". In this case of the throat, the energy manages the communication of the spiritual part with the physical part, that is, the throat controls the insights of the spiritual world and their expression to the physical world. Therefore, there will be no problems in this *chakra*, if the person expresses himself/herself (verbally or non-verbally) according to his/her intuition, values, beliefs and ideals. However, if this expression is not consistent with the "spiritual self", that person will have problems such as difficulty in speaking, severe coughing, difficulty in eating food, problems with the thyroid and feeling of "hairball". We can also have a person who even on hot days puts a scarf around the neck. Everything to protect the energy centre.

The *third eye chakra* is located slightly above the eyes and is associated with the colour indigo blue. It is the energetic centre of intuition, of "seeing further". It is what aggregates the "divine" information and all the information about our existence and experience and helps us in decision making. Any problem in this *chakra* will result in difficulty making decisions, solving problems and emotional and mental instability. It is not surprising that we see people rubbing their noses or scratching their foreheads when they are faced with obstacles to which they cannot find an answer or solution. It is a pleasant way for the body to massage the area that most needs attention. It is extremely common to find these gestures.

Finally, the *crown chakra*. This is located on the top of our head and is associated with the colour violet or white. This energy centre is what connects us to "Heaven". It is the link to other "knowledge plans", it is the link to the "Universal". It is therefore an energy centre linked to wisdom and a high degree of knowledge. It is a mediumship centre. Any problem in this *chakra* will be easily detected by body language: there is a tendency to scratch your head from the top or the back. More specifically in the parietal bones. It is a sign of ignorance or difficulty in finding a path in life or the simple resolution of a pending task. It is usually a *chakra* that articulates closely with the *third eye chakra*. Any problem in these centres, reveals that the person is lacking in inspiration, lack of ideas, lack of solutions and lack of intuition. There may be difficulty in responding to day-to-day requests. It can also reveal a lack of identity or a mission in life.

The purpose of this subchapter was just to mention that the body language combined with the study of the *chakras* helped me a lot in the therapeutic sessions. I was very generic, so I advise you to read more in this field. It will help to understand the body symbolism and what the body transmits to us. I warn that the body is constantly transmitting information to us, whether in therapeutic sessions or outside. Body language is the fastest way to understand this information.

SPIRITISM, PSYCHOGENEALOGY, EXORCISM AND NEW AGE

What do Spiritism, psychogenealogy, exorcism and New Age have in common? Probably very little. So why did I include them in the same subchapter? Because, except for psychogenealogy, they are controversial areas and give rise to the greatest negative reactions. They are a prohibited subject in various contexts, but I highlight only one: the Catholicism. I will make it clear from the start, even though it is a taboo subject and "the work of the devil", in the Catholic perspective, that Spiritism helped me to analyse many of the phenomena described in Chapter II. Its concepts opened horizons for me. Studying exorcism too. As for the New Age philosophy, let's say that I am still ambivalent today as to what have helped me. What is New Age? It's all and nothing at the same time.

Let's start with Spiritism. I recently read an article (the source is not very reliable) that described Spiritism as a demonstration of the "Devil" and pseudoscience. The article leads us to view Spiritism as an easy reading of the "Sacred Scriptures", which makes us believe, wrongly, that the world continues beyond death and that we can return to this Earth when we want to reincarnate. Simply put, if each of us makes mistakes, we can always come back here at another time to correct them. It is a way of not taking responsibility for our earthly life. If it goes wrong, well, we'll continue into the next life. I do not entirely agree with the opinion of the author of the article, but I recognize a good purpose. To study Spiritism, we will have to read Allan Kardec's books. To read them, we will have to accept a premise at the outset: there is a physical world and there is a spiritual world. There is the possibility of contact between one world and the other, through the mediumistic abilities of certain people. In the concepts of Spiritism, my type of mediumistic capacity probably is (I am not sure) "magnetism" or "mediumship of healing", that is, the ability to use energy to heal a person. Someone with this capacity may even influence the electrical world around him/her (which is no longer surprising to me, in my case). In addition to magnetism, there are many other mediumistic capacities. There are then capacities that allow people to "see" other planes than the physical (that is, to see "ghosts", or auras, or similar things); "hearing" sounds (voices of "ghosts", for example);

to be intermediaries between the physical and the spiritual plane, writing messages or making drawings of the information received from the spirits; touch an object and access the memories of the owner of that object. There will be many more. You will certainly have noticed names like psychophony, psychography, scrying, pneumography, pneumatophony or poltergeist. The example of the "writing shoulder" in Chapter II, can be framed in one of these (or not). In fact, all the cases described in Chapter II can be framed in some type of phenomenon.

Spiritism leads us to accept that we are evolving spirits and that earthly life is just another stage in a long process of evolution. It leads us to accept that we can get in touch with the spiritual world, either through mediums or even through our "intuition" (a mediumistic ability).

Why did Spiritism help me? When we are faced with situations that go beyond our understanding, it is natural that we have a magical-religious thought and believe in the supernatural. In my case, not that much. I have always been (and continue to be) sceptical and curious, trying to find answers to the experiences I witnessed. Spiritism helped me to broaden the meaning of "parts". These "parts", of which I speak so much throughout this book, always with quotes and more quotes. These quotes have a purpose. It is to name a multitude of things.

> *These "parts" can be: a cell, a memory, an emotion, an illness or a spirit. Or several. Or even physical manifestations of something that is outside of us. Like, for example, having a certain disease, just because a friend of ours had it.*

This type of energy transfer happens. Even today, after everything I witnessed, I ask myself: "Ricardo, do you really believe in the existence of spirits?". The answer to this is easy. Since I had that experience with Sofia (see Chapter II) and other similar situations, I have come to believe in a lot of things. Are they spirits? Maybe yes. Maybe not. Something is. What? I do not know. Where has it ever crossed my mind to perform physical treatments just with my thoughts and without touching the person, being eight meters away? Where has it ever crossed my mind to have people conscious and talking to me (about trivialities), while their bodies moved without any voluntary control? Where did it cross my mind to separate the "conscious" and the "non-conscious"? And talk to the two as if they were different "entities"? A wonderful world, to be sure, but it brought me so many doubts and some scares. To be talking to more than two and three "parts" at the same time? Were three spirits using the same person's body to communicate with me? Maybe yes. In some cases, I just accepted that idea and the results were the best I've had. When my mind doubted more, "pufff"! The result was frustrating. Do you remember the concept of the "internal doctor"? What if this "internal doctor" is a spirit that will help me to treat people? In my mind, I may be constantly asking questions. From my experience, there are some learnings on this topic:

1. The threshold between the "spiritual world" and "mental illness" is blurred.
2. At a certain point in the "championship", I was so confused, and with such a great sense of ignorance, that I went down. After all, many of the manifestations could be mental illnesses. But what are mental illnesses anyway? Phenomena not explained by science? Pharmacology can, in fact, improve a person. At least functionally, in interaction with the outside world. But does it "cure"?

3. There are people who "travel" to past lives and like to describe incredible worlds. I learned an important thing: we need to bring people into today's life and that's where we are going to solve problems. This is where we will become aware of what we need to change in our lives. This is where we learn. In the present. In today's life.
4. What are past lives? Are they really experiences of our spirit, in other times? Or just generational memories, passed down from our ancestors, over time?

When someone hears about past lives, they are immediately interested in knowing who they were, where they went and whether if they were someone famous. The point is that I have rarely encountered "trips" to past lives. The ones I found were very doubtful. They sounded false. Sounded me like an "escape". Escape from pain, from responsibility, from facing problems, from not accepting a personal characteristic or life event. However, I have had cases where people were able to describe situations in detail, which happened before they were born. Symbolic "dull" memories with people shapes. But they were right when they asked other older people (usually their parents) about the issues. When I went to some hypnosis sessions myself, I went to seek memories of my birth. Memories of events of which I was not aware. And that I confirmed with my parents. However, this type of "information retrieval" does not seem to me at all like a "past life", but rather memories that pass from generation to generation: generational memory. What is generational memory? Generational memory is a topic that has French influence, but with another name: psychogenealogy. This area is very interesting, because with it I realized something for which I was not awake. Our life is giving way to a "bigger life", in this case the family. I am grateful to my father for having drawn my attention to this form of analysis.

As health professionals, and not only, we learn to make genograms and ecomaps, in order to visually perceive the relationship between various people with their environment. Usually, we carry out the basic genealogy, of relationships with grandparents, parents, children, siblings, separations, emotional connections between individuals and other things like that. However, psychogenealogy has alerted me to other details, which are more visible as we collect information from past generations. It is a time-consuming task, if we want it to be detailed, but it will bring precious information to understand a person's "role", or "mission". The ideal is to study more than four generations. People are not always able to provide so much information, so we must adapt to whatever is provided to us. With the study of the generations, we will immediately notice repetitive cycles. Right away, in our name. Who gave us the name? Does the name have any repetition in family history? If so, in which generation or generations? Who was responsible for the name given to us? The father or the mother? An uncle or an aunt? A grandfather or a grandmother? Or a great-grandfather or a great-grandmother? Or a friend? Or, who knows, a soap opera or a *telenovela* that influenced the choice of the name? Right by the name, we can start to see repetitive cycles, with the person who gave us that name. Imagine that you have in your genealogy, in the generation of your great-grandfather or great-grandmother, a family member that has the name of Rodrigo. This family member never had children, but it is known that if he did, he would like it to be a boy. The generations pass and, without any conscience, there is a time in the genealogy when a Rodrigo appears. It may be purely coincidental. However, this coincidence is a reason for study, since the probability of this "new" Rodrigo starting a repetitive cycle with the "old" Rodrigo is enormous. For all intents and purposes, we will have to analyse the new member of the family tree with the last generation that gave it its name. It is not surprising that we find many points in common. Psychogenealogy is a world to be explored and I would never be able to analyse in enough detail the potential that this world has. It is essential to use this knowledge to remain open to certain phenomena that happen in our lives. From illnesses, to injuries we make, to separations or unions and lifestyles, there may be several "coincidences" that we will encounter. In fact, it was with psychogenealogy that, with just one session, I solved the problem described in Chapter II – *Cristina and psychogenealogy*.

Exorcism. Hmm! Even the name scares. Well, it's not to scare. Culturally, we are stuck with fantasies that there is a "demon" behind all events and bad behaviour. It may be, but with all the experiences I had, even the most frightening, there was always a positive purpose behind them. I never took with flying objects on my head, nor with angry speeches in Latin or Greek. Even if that had happened, I would never have understood them. Okay, right. I am going to believe that the issue of the LED bulb fusing and giving off intense smoke was a "fluke". I hope!

Studying exorcism was something I had to do, although I didn't even know where to start. The truth is, I was lucky. Around 2010, on public television, there was a documentary about a priest (or former priest) who performed exorcisms. I dissected his speech over and over. I analysed the images that had been recorded. I analysed his speech and the ideas that could be behind it. This priest described the people who contacted him and what are the most common signs of "possession". In some of these signs, I recognized similarities with cases that had crossed with me, the body movement being the most obvious. Other signs were new, like the fact that people speak to him in Latin. If there were common points in the signs or manifestations of "possession", the same could not be said about the way of acting. My focus has always been to see my role as a "mediator" of communication between the "parts". If there is an emotion, or a memory that wants to communicate, it will naturally seek for the means to do so. Usually, it does so through signs and symptoms, but there are not always those who "hear" them. So, when that "part" finds a channel where it can communicate, it sure becomes much more discoverable.

Imagine a person wanting to talk to someone and who only has a cell phone. That person will certainly use that mobile phone to contact someone. Whether to speak or to ask for help. If someone answers? What will be the most likely reaction? It's starting a conversation. What if the person on the other end rejects the call? We repeat it until the receiver answers. Now, make it more concrete, in bodily terms. If a memory or emotion or other "part" is always using the headache (using the body as a "cell phone") to get someone's attention (making the "call"), when you find a "call" receiver, it will certainly express itself. Most of the time, in "cluttered" ways, such as uncoordinated movements, muscle tension, crying, laughing and many other ways. What happens if someone understands that there is a "part" wanting to communicate and prefer to "reject the call"? Believe me... this "part" will become insistent and more visible!

Therefore, this exorcist's approach differs from mine, evidently. If I find a "part" that wants to communicate, I will certainly want to understand it. Talk to it and understand its needs. However, this exorcist did exactly what I thought was strange! "Get out of this body!" or "Shut up forever!" or "That the Holy water expel you from the body!" is unbelievable, in my view. So, if there is an attempt of the "parts" to communicate, an attempt that has already somatised (to give reasons to call an exorcist), will we prefer to "answer the call" and communicate? Or do we prefer to "hang up the call" and pretend that none of it exists? If you choose the latter case, I believe you will be much more frightened, as the physical manifestations will be much greater. It's like having a pot of boiling water with the lid on. The pressure will increase until it explodes. So... suggestion!

Be a communicator and not an exorcist.

I recently met a psychiatrist who was reading a book on exorcism. He simply wanted to better understand this "world" in order to be able to balance it with his scientific knowledge. In fact, a world with tenuous limits and not always clear. I admire his insight. I also had to read a book on exorcism and chose an author who addresses historical concepts – *spirit possession and exorcism: history, psychology and neurobiology* – and how they evolved in different societies. This book was important to clarify concepts and to understand its importance throughout history. I learned something about empathy.

"The capacity of empathy is the requisite foundation for spirit possession.".

Patrick McNamara

With that psychiatrist, I shared some of my therapeutic "findings". The "treatment at a distance" is the *ex libris*. I told him that my life had changed a lot, that I had been forced to collect myself in the "rabbit hole" and go down to the earth again. He asked me in amazement: "Why?". The reason is simple! Society does not want to know (or is afraid) of what is hidden or that isn't palpable and touchable. This book is being written seven years after my peak of discoveries. Because I was never able to name the "things" I did and do. Because the label of "sorcerer", or "wizard" is quickly taken out of the pocket and placed on our forehead.

Anyway, whenever I could, publicly, even in scientific circles, I made a point of saying that we are losing a "world" of therapeutic potential. I hope someone is curious enough to explore it further.

I remember people traveling more than three hundred kilometres to come to me, because they had good references. Most of them thought that I was a *Harry Potter*, psychic medium or sorcerer, with a "magic wand" that would take their problems away in a few minutes. I don't see myself in this form of therapy, but I understand that it passes that image. Performing body movements without touching the person? Ouch!

New Age. It's a "bullshit" philosophy. It is an "all and nothing" in one thing. It is a series of cliché phrases and independent thinkers that make a "soup" of oriental, western philosophy, personal development, quantum physics, psychology, cosmology, astrology, astronomy and other areas that can be remembered. Naturally, what will come out of there is not a "soup", but probably a very strange mud. Worst of all: New Age entered in the society and in our minds in a fast and cloaked way. It became difficult to discern the relevant from the irrelevant. To make matters worse, it decided to incorporate coaching and neuro-linguistic programming techniques into its repertoire. "Happiness" is a state, it is not a permanent condition or an objective, as we are made to believe. If the "personal goal" is to "be happy", then the "broth is spilled" right away.

(New Age) Stop it, please! You're making too much noise!

IDEOMOTOR REFLEXES, APPLIED KINESIOLOGY AND RADIESTHESIA

I will not go into much detail on this subchapter, as I do not even know very well what to say about these topics. I don't even know if I'm using the right terms. So why dare I talk about them? Because it is important to be aware that "this" exists and that it will bring important information to the therapy. I admit that I may have misunderstood the original concepts, but the way I interpreted them brought me results.

I read that the ideomotor reflexes (or ideomotor effect) would have appeared in the late 18th century and early 19th century. I don't know if it is a coincidence that Spiritism arose at this time. The ideomotor reflexes arose at a time when the "hidden" and the *Ouija board* were being studied a lot. In fact, the first time I got to know this board was around the age of fifteen. From what I heard, my colleagues used it as a kidding to talk to "ghosts" or to the "dead". They put letters and numbers on a table, sat around that table and each put a finger on a glass. From what they said, the glass moved and answered questions that were asked. At this point, at my fifteen years, the discussion of Nostradamus' book and the theories of the end of the world were in fashion. Certainly, when reading about this you must be thinking something like this: "Yes! I know what it is, and I also did it in childhood. I got scared and never again!". I meet a lot of people who have already played these "games". As a teenager, I tried twice, but I never got results. I gave up. Around the age of 28, I came across with colleagues who had been "playing" with this game and had a bad time for a few days. I don't know what happened.

Anyway, what interests me is talking about the ideomotor reflexes. These reflexes are nothing more than involuntary movements of the body. What are they worth for? To give us answers. "Ah, but that is the power of self-suggestion," I am often told. Yes, fine, but what is it anyway? The power of believing? Of faith? What energy is it that seems to work? Can the health professional use it for example with a person who has cancer? "Look… tomorrow, when you wake up, you will no longer have cancer. There is an invisible force that is working on you and tomorrow it will be completely healed.". Is it like this? Unfortunately, not. This "self-suggestion power" has limited action. The ideomotor reflexes are reflexes of a person. Micro-movements that give us an answer. Yes, they are also the basis of dowsing (forgive me dowsing scholars! I know that you have an exhaustive training program and that I am going to be very reductive). Dowsing is what allows people to walk with a "stick" looking for water veins. It works. Ideomotor reflexes are something I use often and rarely fail. In fact, I don't remember of them failing. Still, I always warn people that these methods are fallible.

Ideomotor reflexes use conditioning – which can be done verbally or mentally. We return to the incredible things. The thought to communicate with the other person's "non-conscious". Usually, I prefer to speak, even though I know that what I say may seem ridiculous. To quickly obtain information from the "non-conscious", I use some techniques:

1. The technique of waiting for the person's involuntary movement.
2. The technique I call "applied kinesiology".
3. The pendulum.

Starting with the first technique: waiting for the voluntary movement of the person's body to the questions I ask. When I use this technique, I usually work with three types of possible answers to questions. The questions must be asked in a simple and unambiguous way. It is enough to have more than one interpretation, for the results to go wrong. The ideal is to always test with counter questions. So, my usual codes are:

1. A "yes" is any involuntary movement on the person's right side.
2. A "no" is any involuntary movement on the person's left side.
3. An "I'm not allowed to ask the question" or "I'm not sure" is any involuntary movement in the nose. Usually, in the form of an intense itching in the nose.

To give an example of what it will be like to work in a simple way with the ideomotor reflexes:

1. Lay the person down on a massage table or bed or couch. The person may have his/her eyes open or not. Ask the person to remain still. As still as possible.
2. Verbally (yes, here it is verbally), define that we are going to speak to a "part" that wants to communicate, be it a disease, or organ, or another. It will always depend on the anamnesis we did previously. After all, why did the person come to us?
3. Inform this "part" that any involuntary movement on the right side will correspond to a "yes" and any involuntary movement on the left side will be a "no" and that the itchy nose is a sign of "I am not authorized to do the question "or" I'm not sure ".
4. Start with the question: "Am I allowed to speak to the 'part'?" or "Am I allowed to speak to the internal doctor?" or something like that.
5. Wait for involuntary movements. The minimum movement corresponds to the pre-defined response. Unless it is a

movement that is visibly voluntary. The voluntary movements are well noticed. The involuntary movements are almost always super-fast, sometimes in the form of tremulous and sometimes they frighten the very person who is on the massage table.

6. It is good to be aware of the whole body, waiting for involuntary movements. As a practical matter, I usually limit the movement to the hands: "Any movement of the right hand will be a 'yes', any movement of the left hand will be a 'no'.".

7. The answer is rarely "no". When it is "no", we can repeat the question again, adding "is there anybody who is a better therapist to treat this 'part'?". It is normal for the answer to be yes. If so, we can ask which of the professions fits best: medicine, nursing, physiotherapy, psychology, nutrition, among others. We can ask much more than that, for example, which of the therapies best suits the case.

8. The answer being "yes", will give permission for other questions.

9. In addition to allowing questions, it is customary to have permission for other situations, such as distance treatment.

It sounds simple, but it is not. This phase of obtaining permission can take anywhere from one second to several minutes. In the latter case, we begin to doubt our own techniques and approaches. It takes patience. Which I don't always have. So, I move on to approach number two: "applied kinesiology".

This "applied kinesiology" approach does not seem to have anything to do with what I read about "kinesiology". The science that studies movement is closely linked to manual therapy. Why do I call it "applied kinesiology"? Because I learned that term from an osteopathic colleague who used the muscles to obtain information from the body. How? He pressed trigger points to test the strength of a muscle or organ. Well then. Yes, trigger points exist in manual therapy. This colleague of mine did something else, which is very similar to physical tests for the psoas iliac. Standing or lying down, he asked people to stretch their upper limbs. Then he compared the symmetry of the fingers of both hands. Whether they were aligned or misaligned. Then he would touch a trigger point and compare again. If it was very misaligned, it was because the structure connected to that trigger point needed correction. When I saw this, I thought: "Ricardo, this concept is very interesting. What if instead of touching trigger points, you simply ask questions in your mind?". I started to do it and the body started to answer me. So, I moved on to another type of "parameterization". Any alignment of the thumb nails is a "yes". Any misalignment is a "no". Although this parameterization pleased me, it didn't become practical. I started to notice that people answered me differently. I thought it was due to physical limitations. So, I just started asking the question (most of the time, in my mind, because it is much faster. Rarely, orally): "Body, please give me a yes". "Body, please give me a no". Then, I compared the alignment of the thumb nails and already knew what the body's response was (illustration 7). I must say that this technique is very fast. It almost always works. I say "almost always", because in some cases I was unable to apply it. There are other ways to use the body to answer me. Once, just for testing, I asked a person's body (just in my thinking), to lose the strength of the lower limbs, for the "yes". That man started to descend slowly and asked me for a chair, because he was not feeling well. I immediately asked the body to regain strength. What was my surprise... it was immediate!

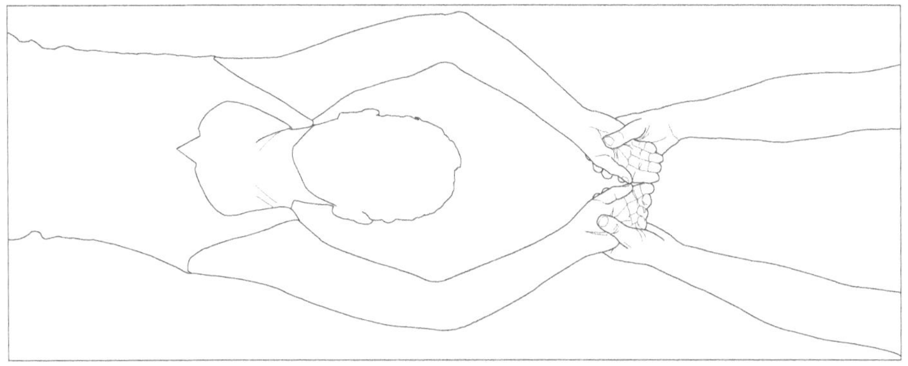

Illustration 7 – "Yes" and "no" tests, comparing the alignment of the thumbs.

I still use this technique a lot today. I have used it enough to know the gender of a child who is still in the womb. Pregnant women are always curious. I have never failed the genre, although I always inform that there is a likelihood of making a mistake. What else can you do? You can immediately communicate with the foetus: "What name do you prefer?", "What do you need from your mother?", "How are you feeling?". All these questions will obviously have to be answered through more questions. For example, to find the preferred name, I must go through the entire alphabet. There are always letters that will give a "strong", "yes" sign. Others that will be weaker. For example, if I give a strong sign on "A", I can ask for names beginning with that letter: "Anabela?", "Alberto?", Andreia? ".

Although the techniques mentioned above are the ones I use the most, there was also a time when I became interested in dowsing (in a very amateur perspective). I bought a pendulum (I still have it), to demonstrate, in a more visual way, the power of the word on the body. The pendulum shows us how our bodies react to each thought. The muscles act unconsciously to our thoughts. I just have a pendulum in my hand, imagine that it goes around in circles, clockwise, that voilá. The pendulum starts to accomplish what was thought. The pendulum was very useful for teaching all people who had "loose" and unclear thoughts. When there was no goal, the pendulum was in a disorderly motion. The pendulum allows us to set parameters other than "yes" and "no". It allows circles in both directions and it allows oscillating movements in a longitudinal and a transverse plane. Allow diagonals. It allows to be stopped. For each of the movements, we can parameterize other issues. "I want a circular movement, clockwise, in case the "X" muscle needs to be treated", "I want an oscillating movement, in the transversal direction, if there is a disease in the "Y" body region", and so on.

OTHERS

Other areas of knowledge helped me to understand more about body symbology: graphology and sophrology. I take the opportunity to add two other areas, which contributed little or nothing: reiki and therapeutic touch.

I started my training in graphology in 2012 and haven't finished it yet. But it will happen soon! I didn't finish it because I have serious difficulties in graduating online. The problem is that in graphology there are many schools, mostly in the United States of America and the United Kingdom. There are also differences between them: the school of "strokes", which only analyses writing for its mechanical component and the school of "strokes" and Gestalt. I chose the second approach. Although I have not yet completed the training, the little I learned was already a lot. Right from the start, the symbology of writing is very similar to that of the body, which

I have already described. The analysis of the sheet as our world, the way we fill it with letters and words, the management of space and margins, the space between letters and between words, strength, energy, inclination and emotional analysis. So many interesting things! Graphology is not considered a science. However, many companies and forensic institutes use it both for the analysis of workers' profiles and for drawing criminal profiles. Just by analysing the writing, we can get a lot of information about the person. It is an unconscious act and, just for that reason, it will give us information that is not always coincident with what the person transmits or wants to transmit.

Sophrology. The name still confuses me, even though I already have some years of knowledge of the therapy. I learned about sophrology through my father, who remembered going to France for training. For some years, I had this training in mind, as I appeared as a kind of "goddess" in the field of psychology and in the field of sport. The focus: breath control. Sophrology can be defined as the study of consciousness and its modifications. Sophrology studies: modified states of consciousness and the means to produce the changes. Uses: breathing exercises; passive or active techniques, derived from hypnosis; the suggestion; traditional relaxation methods, such as *Schultz Autogenic Training*. The truth is that sophrology is a therapy that "drinks" from many sources. One of them I immediately identified: the hypnosis scripts, based on Milton Erickson. Those scripts are so familiar to me. I have talked about this subject before, so I will go ahead. Sophrology never became fashionable in Portugal. I even admit that people who know it are rare. However, they know other modalities of relaxation and well-being, as they have become fashionable and an answer to all ailments. For example? Mindfulness. Remember what I said about New Age?

Let's talk about reiki and the therapeutic touch. Two areas that cause me some discomfort. I get angry. My irritation happens for two reasons: for being fashionable and for not adding knowledge. I am often asked if what I am doing is reiki. No! It's not reiki! I also don't know how to give it a name, because it is a combination of several knowledges, but from reiki has little or nothing. Reiki and therapeutic touch place the hands in various places on the body. To perform the *listening* (see in the previous chapters), I also need to place my hands in various places on the body. It's normal! Does it coincide with the reiki locations? In many cases, yes, but this is perfectly normal. The human body is not immense and infinite. It has limits. There is not much to be invented by hand placement. In vocational training, to my students, I usually put an image of three therapies side by side: fascial therapy, sacro-cranial therapy and reiki. The position of the hands is the same. The same! The concept of each is completely different. In order to (legitimately) be able to criticize reiki, I had to do training in reiki. Just to prove what I already knew. Reiki is the same as giving a pen to a student, before a test for which he/she has not studied, telling him/her that the pen will bring him/her knowledge and allow him/her to have the maximum result: the A. First: knowledge does not come from heaven. It does not arise from spontaneous generation. It requires work. Study. Mistake. Trial and error learning. How can anyone believe that, when doing reiki training (an average of 6 hours per level), they will have healing skills? Because reiki teaches you to make sacred symbols mentally and with your hands and that will heal the person? Seriously? Is it not a principle of not taking responsibility for learning itself? From the suffering that learning brings? Yes, learning does not always bring pleasure. It takes effort. Of course, most people who look for reiki, feel "warm". It doesn't take much for that. It is enough to place another person without training in reiki, with the hands in the same places, without any knowledge of symbols, to obtain the same results. Do I get indignant? Yes. Especially when I know that there are other therapies that bring results and that are discredited because they use techniques "similar to the placement of hands" in reiki. It's fashion. I understand. What I don't understand is how someone believes they will have supernatural powers just because they learned symbols. For this, it is better to bet on religions. They have a lot more symbols, a lot more rituals, mantras and mandalas. Then, we have another fashion, which comes from New Age (again New Age). There is a reiki fashion, which is to communicate with beings from other planes of existence, namely with reptiles – the "reptilians" – who command all our thoughts and actions. Or, that a muscular contracture is an extra-terrestrial "chip", to control us from a distance.

Thus, it is difficult to innovate in health and explore new fields. We will always remain in the obvious therapy: the one we are able to manipulate. Never in life will we study how it is possible to create physical movement, at a distance, with thought. If this exist, there must be an explanation. It must be understood, in order to be replicated. We must know the principles by which this happens. So that we don't always walk around in "trial and error".

The therapeutic touch was something I learned in my nursing degree, when I was nineteen. I thought that was "bullshit". Put my hands on a person's head so that he/she could feel warm? Hmm. As I currently see it, the therapeutic touch does have potentials, but they are underused. Very underused.

Let's be curious! In neurolinguistic programming, we summarize learning in a simple way, using the TOTE: Test; Operate; Test; Exit.

The same is to say:

1. Test.
2. Does it work? No.
3. Retest.
4. Does it work? No.
5. Then, retest.
6. Does it work? Yes.
7. Then leave.
8. The learning is done.

PERSONAL NOTES AND GUIDELINES

In this subchapter, I will conclude with some ideas that helped me to understand the world. I admit that they may not be scientifically correct, but they have become good allies. It is true that some came under the influence of New Age, which I criticize so much.

THE INFINITELY BIG AND THE INFINITELY SMALL

I have always spoken of "parts" and "non-conscious" in this book. Always with quotes. The "parts" and the "non-conscious" can be everything. Now, we contextualize these "parts" from what we know of the universe. We have universes at various levels. In quantum physics, we admit the existence of the subatomic world. We were able to identify structures under the microscope. Each with a function. Our body is made up of several cells, which make up tissues, organs, systems and, in the end, give a complete organism. This organism functions as a "part" of a larger organism – the family. Not only family, but groups of people, communities, regions, countries, continents. In the end, another organism: the planet Earth. This planet that is in the middle of a vastness of other "beings". Have you noticed that the atom scheme and the representation of the electron movement is very similar to the representation of the Solar System? And our galaxy? What if we are just "subatomic" particles in an organism? What if inside of us, we also have this number of universes? Confused? Perhaps. Just to say that when I speak of "parts" it is to have the idea that this can represent things of which we are not even aware. If you prefer, you can be specific to the point you know. Do you want to talk to a cell's "Golgi complex"? Do it.

We have universes within us, and we are also part of larger universes. See the end of the *Men in Black* film trilogy and you will have a visual aid. Or imagine the Russian dolls, the *matryoshkas*.

THE MECHANICS OF PHYSICAL AND EMOTIONAL TRAUMA

There are several trauma books. In medicine, this trauma has a very concrete definition. However, my idea of "trauma" changed when I read that concept from an osteopathic perspective. Although the theory remained in physical perspective, we can translate it into emotional trauma. The concepts are related to mechanics and energy. Forgive me, physicists (which I know will present me entire textbooks on physics and say that I am just saying nonsense), but I will explain the concepts in a simplistic way.

Let's start from a simple example. Hot water has a lot of kinetic energy (from moving particles). This energy will pass to systems with lower energy (in this case, cold water). Every day we work with this concept, mainly in the kitchen. Do you want to warm your child's milk mug? You place it in a water bath, with hot water outside. Right? Because there will be a thermal balance. Hot water will lose energy. Cold milk will capture energy. It will warm up or at least stay warm.

Imagine the same principle in the human body. As I have a lot of experience in the sports world, I will give an example of this area: a football player who gets kicked in the leg. This kick acts as an "injection" of energy into the athlete's body. It is necessary to start from the idea that the body has a limited capacity to absorb energy. In football, we added a barrier that dissipates the entry of that energy: the shin guards. In this case, we will omit the shin guards. The player who takes a kick has a large energy input in the leg. This energy will be dissipated by the body. The impact zone will certainly absorb most of the energy, but the rest will be dissipated to other locations: knee, hip, spine, head, organs, bones, or other structures. Each of these will assimilate that same energy differently. What happens if the energy input is greater than the body's ability to dissipate? In this case, the bone fracture. Or a muscle strain. Therefore, when we talk about the mechanics of trauma, it is necessary to be aware that the lesions have repercussions on the entire body. That is, a sprain can create (and creates) impact on other structures, so a player's headache can come from that same sprain.

The same principle applies to emotional trauma. If we view emotions (*e-motion*) as kinetic energy, we quickly understand "emotional pain". Take the end of a loving relationship as an example. This energy (either in the emotional form or whatever you want to call it) will be captured by the specific organ of that emotion. In this case, the heart. The heart will absorb the energy as much as it can. Some energy will go to other structures, like "dissipation waves". What if the energy exceeds the heart's tolerance capacity? Well, in the extreme, in short, it results in cardiac arrest. It is not a rare case. We often see people die within days of a life partner's death. The heart just stops. We say that he/she died of love, or of heartbreak. So it is, effectively. But let's not just think about the extreme. Think of the middle. An "emotional" energy problem in the heart can result in somatization, such as pain, arrhythmias, bradycardia or tachycardia.

What do I look for as a therapist? I look for places that have accumulated more energy, so I can treat them. See the example I gave in the subchapter of "body language", in the *RTP news*. To some extent, this energy in reserve is what constitutes the "energy cysts" that I spoke of in the book. It must be released before it causes great physical damage.

WAYS OF COMMUNICATION

There are several ways to communicate with the "non-conscious" of the person we are following: by touch, by word, by writing, by mental images (mental pop-ups), dreams and even intuition. To do this, we need to learn to trust this form of communication. We are so focused on the tangible, the objective and the measurable, that we forget the most instinctive part. In these therapeutic cases, it is necessary to relearn the concept of anamnesis and the ways of obtaining information.

In illustration 8, I represent one of the most used techniques for the "first diagnosis" to the "non-conscious". It is a general test, of fascial evaluation, not specific, but that will give me strong indicators of:

1. Possibility of entering a trance, through touch.
2. Expected intensity of the trance.
3. Location of injuries, illnesses or "emotional cysts".
4. Time reference: past, present or future.

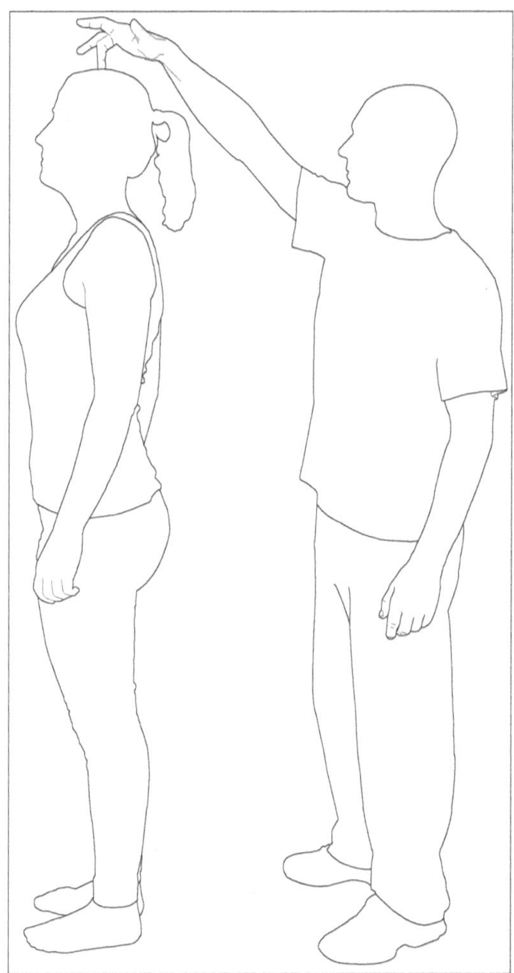

Illustration 8 – Fascial evaluation technique. It is like the technique used in illustration 5, but in which we touch the person, with a finger on the parietal bones.

DO NOT THINK. WAIT!

Over the past eleven years, exploring these new therapeutic forms, the most difficult has not been to see people moving as if they were cases of "exorcism or demonic possession", or doing remote treatments. It was my thought. It took me a long time to re-educate my way of looking at the world and the concepts of "life", "health", "disease" and "health professional". Sceptical, and always oriented towards understanding everything around me, I always tried to find out more about different areas, in search of answers. The setback is that it took a lot of energy and drew attention to my ignorance. There is so much to learn that I felt (feel) tiny and unable to assimilate such knowledge. It took me some time to learn to relativize and accept that I am not "perfect", "immense" and "owner of the truth". So, every time I had a person in front of me, I was anxious. I felt that I had to "give him/her something", because that was his/her expectation. The more I thought I had to have results, the less it happened. I had to learn to give up wanting. Giving up on *listening*, with a whirlwind of theories in mind. I just had to learn to wait for the "non-conscious" response, regardless of the time that took (sometimes, several minutes). There is a very good indicator, but not always present, which is REM (*rapid eye movement*). When I am *listening* (illustration 9), one of the input signals in "trance" is precisely the REM.

"Do not think. Wait for REM!".

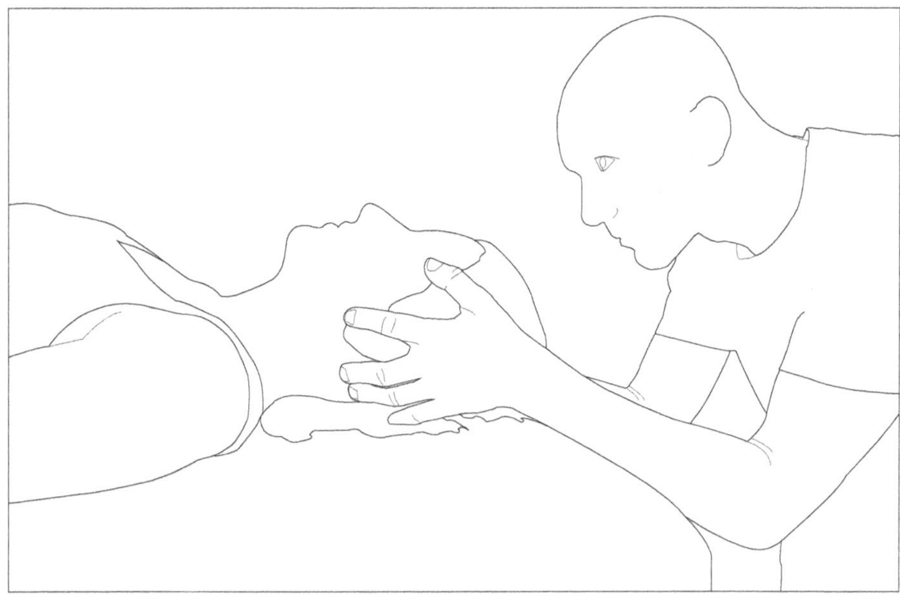

Illustration 9 – Performing *listening*, in my favourite position: at the head of the massage table, with my hands on the person's head, being able to visualize in detail the REM (rapid eye movement), as well as the rest of the body.

DIFFICULTIES IN COMMUNICATING WITH THE "NON-CONSCIOUS" OR WITH THE "PARTS"

It all seems very simple and fabulous from the experiences I have been sharing. The truth is that there is no therapy that suits all people, in all contexts and in all cases. There are several obstacles that I encountered and still encounter, when the subject is related to the communication between "me" and the "parts" or the "non-conscious": disorientation; past, present or future; "free spinning wheel", rejection and resistance; "reset"; with whom I am talking to.

Disorientation is the first obstacle to be overcome. Disorientation appears when someone brings me a problem and informs me of the number of professionals they have been through and the lack of results they have had. "Where to start?". That is why it is important to have several possibilities for analysis, which obviously implies both theoretical and practical knowledge. I usually use ideomotor reflexes and a quick body test, based on some ideas from fascial therapy. It's simple. With the person standing, I place my index finger on the person's head and analyse the body's movement (front, back, loss of strength, oscillations, speed of response, among other movements). This test (illustration 8), will already bring me a lot of information.

Past, present or future. Is the illness or problem that the person presents to me a reflection of the past, is it the present or is it something that has not yet happened? Anxiety is often a symptom of people living in the future. They live with obsessions and concerns in a negative world. Intuition can contribute to this. They are extremely sensitive to the point of being able to predict future events with a high degree of precision. It may not be in a detailed way, but in a symbolic way or in an "overview". Framing the time period is a challenge, not always clear. As a rule, I try to explore the past.

The "free spinning wheel" is the name I give to those sessions in which information appears on all sides, but without much benefit. It is common to happen when there are several "parts" wanting to speak at the same time. The physical manifestations are exuberant, appear from different bodily areas and, when we try to talk to them, the information appears in a disorganized and unrelated way. It can also happen when a "part" wants to say a lot in a very short time. Solution? Be very objective and define that there are rules, such as saying "one at a time" and, if the rules are not followed, the session is ended. It usually works. The imposition of rules is an important condition in this whole process. Reread the case "This is not the way you will communicate", in Chapter II.

Rejections and resistance. The "non-conscious" does not always allow us to ask questions or to do some treatment. Hence, there is a great learning: as therapists, we only act if it allows us. This learning is valid for all physical treatments that we are used to doing. Or for all those moments when we think we are really helping the person. I believe that most of the therapies we do are not having the effect we would like. Reason: we are not the right person to do so, or there is simply no "superior authorization" for this to happen. It's weird, I know. When there are rejections to questions or treatments, we stop there. Everything we do will have no impact. As for the resistances, they depend on the reason. Is the "part" afraid to communicate? Is it a matter of trust? Of fear? Before starting a session, we must make sure that there is full confidence, otherwise we will not get results.

The "reset" is one of the bodily manifestations that I like the most. It is the "letting down of the guard" that allows us almost all types of interventions: speaking, creating movement with thought, asking the "internal doctor" to proceed with self-correction, and much more. Unfortunately, it is not always possible to create this "reset." It is not in our control. It is also a physical manifestation that can be frightening. Suddenly, the person may even be "absent" for a few seconds. The person may be cold or pale or even stop breathing. Fortunately, all of this lasts a few seconds and the persons who experienced it may experience significant improvements in the signs and symptoms that made them seek help. So, in a "simple" way.

Finally, I draw attention to situations in which we do not know with "what" or "with whom" we are communicating. At certain times, I doubted I was talking with a disease, or a cell, or organ, or some body structure. The "part" or the "parts" looked like people. Several people talking at the same time. With its own thought, its own rhythm of conversation and a different lexicon. Emotionally, they appeared to be quite distinct entities. If I followed the perspective of Spiritism, I would be able to explain it: they were different spirits, using the same communication channel. I prefer to remain more sceptical and consider that there are emotions, or memories, or "emotional cysts", in different areas of the body, which are eager to share information. So, do it in an orderly manner. Once again, it is necessary to create rules of communication.

If you ever have an experience like those described in Chapter II, I would like to call your attention to some caution in dealing with diseases such as cancer. Cancer carries immense energy and is like a "part" that is boycotting the entire system. For ethical reasons, I have not yet risked exploring the potential of this form of therapeutic approach. I don't want to give false hope to people who have cancer. I prefer that they follow conventional therapy. I will only accept trying to communicate with this disease (considering it as a "part") if the person unequivocally expresses to me that this is his/her desire and that he/she will continue with conventional therapy. I believe that a great deal of negotiation power is needed with a disease of this kind, based on reports I read from the creator of sacro-cranial therapy. The right time will come to risk doing so.

ADVICE TO HEALTH PROFESSIONALS

I am a health professional with extensive experience in manual therapy. I also have a scientific background. I have a master's degree and I am currently completing my PhD. I know the potential of science. I also know many of its flaws. Science helps us to discover what we have not yet discovered. For that, it is necessary to dare to explore the unknown. Most of the experiences that I described in Chapter II changed my view of "life", "health" and "disease" and made me reflect on my role as a professional. Resistance to these topics – "hidden", as many will call it – takes us away from knowledge. It makes us just one more sheep in the flock.

Dear health professional, I ask you to contemplate therapeutic alternatives different from those taught in the university and in scientific articles. If my generation, and the generations that precede me, are resistant to change, it will be up to the energy of the youngest to dare to continue the work.

I conclude this book with two quotes from the actor Anthony Hopkins, in the film The Rite.

"The interesting thing about sceptics and atheists is that we are always looking for proof, certainty. The question is: what on earth would we do if we found it?".

"Choosing not to believe in the devil won't protect you from him.".

www.ingramcontent.com/pod-product-compliance
Lightning Source LLC
Chambersburg PA
CBHW021955120726
47992CB00001B/272